HEART
TO
HEART

HEART TO HEART

A GUIDE TO THE PSYCHOLOGICAL ASPECTS OF HEART DISEASE

By Herbert N. Budnick, Ph.D.
with Scott Robert Hays

Foreword by
Benjamin Rosin, M.D.

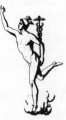

Health Press
Santa Fe, NM 87504

Published by Health Press
P.O. Drawer 1388
Santa Fe NM 87504

ISBN 0-929173-15-5

Library of Congress Cataloging-in-Publication Data

Budnick, Herbert N.
Heart to Heart

1. Coronary Heart Disease -- Psychological Aspects. I. Title.
RC685.C6B83 1990   616.1'23'0019--dc20   90-4737

Printed in the United States of America
10 9 8 7 6 5 4 3 2

Cover Design by Joanna Hill
Heart Illustrations by Danette Rowe
Diagram by John Inserra

ACKNOWLEDGEMENTS

♡ My wife, Ceese, for her numerous ideas and marketing expertise; her sacrifice and support enabled me to realize my vision.

♡ All the cardiac patients and their spouses who allowed me to share in their pain; and Evan McCabe, RN, who encouraged me to "spread the word."

♡ My brother Martin with whom I share a family history of cardiovascular disease.

♡ The cardiac rehab staff at Torrance Memorial Hospital (Barbara, Jennifer, Judy, Mitzy) and the cardiac rehab staff at Little Company of Mary Hospital — for their support and friendship. Also the cardiologists who have supported my efforts and consulted with me over the years.

♡ The Mended Hearts Club for their interest in my work.

♡ The American Heart Association, Los Angeles Chapter, for their assistance and for their work with cardiac patients.

♡ My friends, who encouraged me throughout the writing period, particularly Jeff Balsam.

♡ Toni Rabinowitz for her on-going caring and support, and Don Saracco for his friendship and professional stimulation.

♡ My agent, Linda Chester, for her continued belief and interest in the book, and my publisher, for taking a personal interest and making the "process" enjoyable.

♡ Scott Hays, for his writing ability as well as his caring, understanding and patience.

♡ And finally, the "Neighbors."

To my father, Aaron, and my sister, Rhoda,
both of whom died of cardiovascular disease.

TABLE OF CONTENTS

Chapter Six continued

Cardiovascular disease is indiscriminate. It does not distinguish between male or female. In fact, of the 1.5 million new cases each year, roughly 250,000 of them (16.6%) are women. This book is written for heart disease patients of both sexes, but because of sheer numbers it is the male gender that is referenced in the text, and the general approach is designed for the male cardiac patient with a wife and children. Because there are certain issues which only affect women, there are brief overviews in Chapter Three and Four of those issues which are characteristic of female cardiac patients.

Cardiac patients without a built-in familial support system must reach out to friends, co-workers, or other relatives, for the physical and emotional support essential to recovery.

Actual situations and the experiences of real people were the basis for the examples cited in this book. However, the names have been changed to protect privacy. In some instances, the cases cited are composite creations based on the author's professional experience.

This book expresses the opinions of the authors, and is not intended to replace the services of a physician or a psychologist. Any medical recommendation should be evaluated thoroughly with an individual's personal physician, with suitable consultation as needed.

If in reading through the questions and answers in *Heart to Heart* and participating in the exercises, you experience some emotional distress, you may wish to seek professional help.

FOREWORD

During the late 1950s, when I first entered the field of cardiology, patients with myocardial infarction were confined to hospital beds for extended periods of time. It was generally assumed that their illness marked an end to a productive life, or that their lifestyle would be drastically restricted. Then, the medical profession could offer little that would reduce the risk of a fatal outcome.

Today's patients of acute myocardial infarction are often home to recuperate within days of a heart attack or surgery. Doctors now encourage patients to participate in rehabilitation programs. Thanks to remarkable advances in cardiovascular therapy, a great number of individuals are not only surviving heart attacks but are achieving a far more active and healthy lifestyle.

Along with these remarkable advances in medical and surgical treatment of coronary artery disease, it has also become evident that demanding psychological and social adjustments can have a tremendous impact on future myocardial infarction, cardiac arrhythmias, and the risk of sudden cardiac death. Further impact is felt in recovery and in life expectancy.

Quality of life is built on psychological and social well-being, thus making these factors an integral part of cardiac treatment.

Families affected by heart disease must learn to deal with drastic changes in their lifestyle. They must learn to plough through the five phases of abandonment: helplessness, anger, depression, anxiety and frustration. Having an understanding of these emotional dynamics of heart disease often leads to a speedier and smoother recovery.

For the past ten years, Dr. Budnick has worked in the trenches of the cardiac rehabilitation program at Torrance Memorial Medical Center. He has developed and directed training programs for our medical and nursing staff, focusing on the problems associated with difficult and emotionally distraught cardiac patients.

Dr. Budnick has offered counseling on everything from dietary and lifestyle changes to the need for coronary angioplasty. His "Living With Heart Disease" program has lifted the spirits of countless patients and their families.

Over the years I have had the opportunity to evaluate the effectiveness of his intervention, measured by a reduction in both anxiety and depression. Furthermore, physiological changes were often affected by reduction in tachycardia, blood pressure, and arrhythmias, which are often anxiety induced.

Heart to Heart provides all of us with a wealth of information about the emotional dynamics of heart disease, and provides immediate benefit to the conflicting emotions shared by so many patients and their families.

Benjamin Rosin, MD, Director of Cardiology
Torrance Memorial Medical Center

INTRODUCTION
ORIGINAL EDITION, 1991

When I think back to my childhood, a time that should be remembered as warm and nurturing, all I have are cold, distant impressions. Details from this particular period of my life are sketchy, mostly because I have somehow blocked from memory a very painful reality — the traumatic effect of my father's four heart attacks on me and my family.

The year was 1954 and the place was my parents' home in an upper middle-class neighborhood of Rockville Center, New York. My father, Aaron Budnick, was a hardworking man in his late 40s who did well for himself as a clothing manufacturer. Work had always been a priority in his life; his family came second. And for what he lacked in compassion he tried to make up in charity. He was a strict disciplinarian with a hair-trigger temper who would occasionally threaten corporal punishment with a large leather belt. My mother, Phoebe, played the role of caretaker and mediator. Her life revolved around my father's life and six years after he died, she died of a lonely heart.

At the time of my father's first heart attack, my older brother Martin and older sister Rhoda were away at college. I was left alone, with my mother, to bear the burden of my father's recuperation period, a time of conflicting emotions for all of us.

My confusion stemmed from the fact that no one ever explained to me the extent of my father's illness, why he had suffered a heart attack, and how it would affect our family. My mother would speak in whispers when I entered the room or send me upstairs while she conferred with the doctors and nurses. I felt ignored, and eventually I felt responsible for my father's condition (most children who are left in the dark about their parent's illness feel responsible).

I also can remember as a young boy feeling lonely and rejected by my parents during the years of my father's illness. Although we were never an extremely close family, we did share some good times. But after my father's first heart attack, living at home was like living alone.

My father was never an emotionally giving person. After his first heart attack, a rather serious one which killed a large percentage of his heart muscle, he became self-absorbed, depressed and extremely angry at those he loved the most. The mere fact that everyone was *doing* for him made him believe that he could no longer *do for himself*. He had come to identify himself by what he could give others. When he could no longer give, he gave up.

One rather vivid memory I have is of my father — a broken, defeated man — lying in a hospital bed with tubes and conduits running from his body to a life-support system. His face was pallid and gaunt, and I remember thinking, "This is not the way I want to remember my father." And yet that is exactly how I remember him.

My mother, the ever-present caretaker, neglected her own needs to take care of my father's, and she resented him for it. My father, who needed nurturing, resented my mother's role as caretaker. During one rather strained period, my father was having difficulty urinating. When finally he was able to relieve himself, he called my mother in to help. She rightly told him not to worry about it and go ahead. I could see the devastation on his face as he wet the bed linen. The next day I trembled with fear while he berated my mother over some insignificant issue. His hostility, I later learned, was the direct result of mounting frustrations over his inability to do for himself.

My mother always took the abuse because she feared that challenging him would only exacerbate his condition. Having my own set of frustrations, I withdrew to my own little world. My mother eventually turned to me to fill the emotional void that existed in her life. By the end of the year, each of us had redefined our roles within the family unit.

The expectations we had of each other also changed. Dad and I no longer played catch in the backyard. He could barely walk. My mother took a job at a dry cleaners. We eventually moved to Florida so my father could look for a new job. One year later we moved back to New York. After the second and third heart attacks, my father's condition deteriorated rapidly.

When he finally died at the age of 52, six years after his first heart attack, I felt relieved. I had become so alienated from him and bitter about his illness that it was like watching a stranger being buried. I don't even remember crying at his funeral. But I do remember asking myself, "Why did this happen to me?"

A heart attack occurs when a supply of blood to the heart muscle is severely reduced or halted because of an obstruction in one of the coronary arteries (the arteries that supply blood to the heart muscle). Disability or death can result, depending on how much of the heart muscle is damaged. The American Heart Association estimates that one in four Americans suffer from cardiovascular disease, primarily heart attacks.

Treatment for heart disease was drastically different during my father's time. Rest was the prescribed cure-all, bypass surgery was a fantasy, cardiac rehabilitation centers were nonexistent, and medical equipment was less than adequate. Thanks to biochemical and technological advances in the medical industry — and a far better understanding of psychological factors related to heart disease — nearly two-thirds of today's heart attack victims survive.

Although physical inactivity has never been clearly established as a risk factor for heart disease, many doctors recognize the importance of exercise. To that end, most of the 6,000 general hospitals in the United States have coronary care programs.

But of the major risk factors associated with heart disease — genetics, cigarette smoking, high blood pressure, high cholesterol levels, stress and diabetes — most physicians ignore the psychological factors that lead to, say, stress or high blood pressure, primarily because they are not trained or educated in this particular field. Those who are schooled in psychology typically don't have the time to offer counseling. In fact, few hospitals around the country have adequate psychological counseling programs for the cardiac patient, although they do provide referral services and some in-house counseling sessions.

The fine-tuning of complex and demanding psychological and social adjustments are just as imperative as medical supervision. In fact, a better understanding of these factors actually may lead to a quicker recovery. Hence, it is imperative that a family find answers to the myriad of questions that arise during this medical crisis.

Only a few books, if any, on the market today address the psychological aspects of heart disease, and most of these offer only superficial advice. *Heart to Heart* is written specifically for the cardiac patient and his or her family. It is not written as a guide to self-treatment, but as a thorough reference work on the many aspects of heart disease.

Heart to Heart attempts to answer those questions that have been asked of me by my patients and their families over the last ten years. Naturally, this book can't possibly provide every answer to every question about heart disease. But it can provide the reader with a solid foundation from which to learn more about yourself, your family and this debilitating disease. I also believe the material found in this book can be a useful tool for all health professionals in the medical industry.

With proper counseling, patients and their families need not experience the emotional turmoil that I experienced as a young child. My family was devastated by my father's four heart attacks. I just hope this book will help other families understand the psychological dynamics of heart disease more completely and, ultimately, help ease their journey through the chaos and confusion.

— H. Budnick, Ph.D.

INTRODUCTION
SECOND EDITION, 1997

Since the publication of *Heart to Heart* in 1991 there has been a revolution in health care. Certainly, the managed care movement has been an integral component of this revolution. But, it has been the new focus on the psychological aspects of heart disease and other illnesses that has brought a new dimension to treatment and placed more responsibility on the patient for his/her recovery.

The American Association of Cardiovascular Pulmonary Resuscitation (AACVPR) published new guidelines for cardiac rehabilitation programs in 1996. These guidelines suggest that each program provide for the treatment of the psychological aspects of heart disease. As a matter of fact, in the years to follow we may see a switch from placing emphasis on the physical aspects of recovery to placing more emphasis on the psychological aspects of recovery. (In South Africa and Australia this has already taken place.)

Extensive research validates the critical importance of emotional support/treatment. Social isolation is now seen as a cardiac risk factor and this has elicited new energy and direction for cardiac rehabilitation programs as well as for those professionals who work with cardiac patients and their families. Without question, treating the patient in isolation of those around him/her is to omit a vital recovery component which just may increase the probability of further cardiac difficulties.

For example, in 1979 social scientists conducted a study of 7000 people, statistically a significant amount of people. This study conclude that there was a direct relationship between community or social ties and a person's chance of dying from any cause.

In 1984 in the New England Journal of Medicine, arguably the most prestigious medical journal in the United States, social isolation was agin studied. This time in connection with stress. It was found that those cardiac patients with a high degree of stress and who were socially isolated had a four-fold increased chance of experiencing a second heart attack. It should be noted that at least in the initial stages of cardiac recovery most, if not all, patients experience some degree of stress, if only from the illness itself, and some degree of social isolation, since most, if not all, patients turn inward to the point of being insensitive to the needs of those around them.

More recently in the 1990's Dr. Redford Williams, Duke University conducted a study of 1400 heart attack patients. The conclusion was consistent with other research, that is to say, he found that those patients who had neither a spouse nor close friends were three times more likely to die than those involved in a caring relationship. He further concluded that with minimal heart muscle damage there is a 10% death rate over a five year period. For those patients who had social support the death rate dropped to 5% over the same five year period. That's a 50% decrease in death rate!!

For those who were socially isolated the death rate increased to 15%. The figures are even more dramatic for those with sever heart muscle damage. For this group there is a 40% death rate over a five year period of time. For those with a close relationship the death rate dropped to 20%. For those without companionship the death rate increased to 60%.

Obviously, one of the keys to recovery, then, is to develop and maintain a close relationship. Allowing yourself to be open, honest and direct in your communication with others is the foundation for such relationships. Sharing with your spouse and others will help to decrease social isolation and enable you to reach out to others.

Heart to Heart provides the knowledge, tools and sample dialogue to help you develop the closeness you need to reduce the risk factor of social isolation and increase your quality of life.

It is the social and emotional connection we all crave and need. Mother Theresa once said "The great hunger in America is not about food, it is about alienation."

—H. Budnick, Ph.D.

CHAPTER ONE

SCARED AND CONFUSED: THE CARDIAC PATIENT

After my father died, I retreated from society as a means of survival. I suppressed my emotions, pushed friends away, and got caught up in an endless cycle of destructive relationships. By the time I turned 30 I had become, in effect, my father — a lonely, bitter man. Looking back, I think what caused the most damage was my sense of aloneness. I often wonder what life would have been like had my father not suffered four heart attacks.

Over the years I learned to deal with these conflicting emotions. My mettle actually was put to the test in 1986 when my sister Rhoda, 54, died from heart failure complicated by diabetes. One year prior to this, my brother Martin had undergone triple bypass surgery. The anxiety and depression that they experienced were, in part, present because of the many unknowns associated with heart disease.

This book and my "Living with Heart Disease" philosophy are based on clinical experience and a large body of medical and psychological research, all of which stress the importance of dealing with the *behavioral* and *psychological* factors of heart disease.

With proper intervention, patients and their families can lead happy, productive lives. Intervention may come in several forms. At one end of the continuum are the questions and answers you are about to read. They are based on the interchanges I have had with cardiac patients since 1980. At the other end of the continuum are the physicians and psychotherapists who are specifically trained in dealing with the problems associated with cardiac disease. Seek the level of help you need. Don't wait!

IN THE BEGINNING

Why do I feel inadequate?

You've just suffered a serious, life-threatening illness. Naturally, you're worried about your health, your family, and your job. "How will I pay for these medical expenses? Will I be as active as I was before the illness?" These questions and many others are unanswerable, mostly because you are still in the infancy stage of recuperation. In short, you're questioning your ability to be able to perform as you did before your illness.

Because of these unknowns you feel as if you have little or no control over what is happening to you or over your medications and their side effects, vis-a-vis impotency, depression, nausea, confusion, or inability to concentrate.

Remember, the less control you feel the less likely you will be to attempt anything new. As this process continues, your sense of inadequacy will increase. In order to break this cycle you will need to learn as much as possible about the effects of your illness (for you) and begin to attempt to take on more tasks, *with physician approval, of course.* As you continue to have successes your self confidence will build and your sense of inadequacy will decrease.

Why do I feel lost and confused?

A serious heart attack, especially one that has destroyed a large percentage of your heart muscle, will not only change the complexion of your lifestyle, but will also disrupt the inner dynamics of the family unit. Your spouse becomes your caretaker. Your children may pitch in with the housework or get part-time jobs to help pay for medical expenses. You, on the other hand, knowing little about your illness or what lies ahead, feel confused about the present and future. Additionally, you feel lost because at the moment you don't have any direction beyond getting well, and even here control seems to elude you.

But as the crisis passes and you begin to reach out, you'll become more involved in your old activities. With each task that you attempt a new direction will become clearer. As these changes take place, you'll need all the support you can get. This can come from your family, your physician or rehabilitation nurse, or a support group. What is important here is that you seek this kind of help.

Will I ever be the same?

Do you want to be the same person you were before the heart attack? If your lifestyle and personality contributed to your illness, perhaps it's best to explore other alternatives. This may mean learning new ways to cope with life's pressures. You may have to learn to be more open with yourself and others. Learn to put yourself first, your family second and your job third. Change doesn't come easy. But who knows? You may even like the new, healthy you.

THE BIG FOUR: ANGER, FRUSTRATION, ANXIETY AND DEPRESSION

Why am I angry?

Anger is a powerful emotion and a difficult one to control. Serious heart trouble and all the frustrations that go along with it will sometimes make you even angrier. Anger is a natural reaction in the face of losing your lifestyle as you once knew it, even though it may be expressed at inappropriate times and in inappropriate ways.

In time you will learn that nothing will ever be the same. Your self-perception has changed, as has your perception of others. Emotional and behavioral patterns that you developed over a life span are now different. For most of us, it's easier to embrace the emotions of others than to acknowledge our own. However, it's paramount that we openly embrace our own emotions.

It is not the Type A personality who is a prime candidate for heart disease, but the anger associated with the Type A personality that makes one prone to heart disease. Therefore, addressing your anger becomes tremendously important.

Perhaps you feel helpless and frustrated over your current situation. When you suppress your anger and other emotions, it has to find expression elsewhere. Physically it may lead to abdominal difficulties, muscle pains, rashes, headaches, diarrhea, or chest pains. Emotionally, you may experience depression and irritable behavior, which may cause you to lose the ability to concentrate. This is what I've termed the "circular" issues of heart disease, because your inability to concentrate may also lead to further anger.

The key to dealing with these inner conflicts is to accept your current physical and emotional states, and to learn to release anger through the sharing of emotions — before they reach crisis proportions. Talk with friends, relatives or health professionals. Change comes gradually, but eventually it will help you to better cope with your new lifestyle.

Why am I frustrated?

No matter who you are or what position you hold at work, there's always that sense of vulnerability when you've been waylaid with serious heart trouble. You may want to maintain your position at work and eventually live out a pleasant retirement. But when something like a heart attack interrupts that flow, especially if it means you can never go back to your old lifestyle or continue to pursue your old goals, you become frustrated.

Often these frustrations can cause you to feel discouraged and puzzled. The perceived lack of control you have over your environment (family, work, etc.) may cause you to feel anxious and irritable. All of these emotions are interrelated. No single one is separate from the others. Adjust your lifestyle accordingly. Strive only for those goals that you can accomplish. As you begin to become aware of your successes, your self-worth will increase and your frustration will diminish.

Why am I anxious?

Anxiety and depression are natural reactions for a cardiac patient. If you are not experiencing these emotions, you're probably suppressing them — which is counterproductive. Typically, anxiety is seen through physiological signs like

5

sweating and an increased pulse rate. The uncertainty, fear and apprehension you have about your cardiac difficulties may also cause you to feel anxious and worried about the changes in your life. The uncertainties revolve around real and perceived impressions. Perhaps you're worried about suffering another heart attack, or that you'll be physically handicapped for the rest of your life.

Don't push these fears away. Share them with your doctor, your family and with a support group, if needed. In time, as you exert more control over your life, the anxiety will become more manageable.

Why am I depressed?

Depression also is a natural emotional reaction to heart disease. It is present, in part, because of your sense of loss and helplessness. Acknowledging this "circular" pattern — by talking with doctors and nurses — may help you to clear the mystery surrounding your depression.

The thought of making changes in your lifestyle also may depress you, especially if you think you don't have the emotional support of family or friends. Reach out to them anyway. Allow them to help you with decisions and adjustments. It's certainly not going to be easy for them, but it will be easier for all concerned if you work together.

Some of the medication you're taking may also produce some degree of depression. Again, talk to your physician.

In general, a personal inventory of what you can and cannot do in your life may help lessen your depression. Realistically, this process may take six months to a year. With this time frame in mind, recovery is easier to comprehend and setbacks are not as insurmountable.

LIVING WITH HEART DISEASE

How do I learn to cope with my illness?

Coping ultimately involves your ability to be flexible and your desire to change. Look for alternative ways to respond to stressful situations.

To help build your self-confidence, do only those tasks that you can accomplish. Take on small projects around the house. Set aside 15 minutes every day to talk to your spouse or family. Talk about your day, about your relationships, about your illness. This creates a closeness with your family and helps focus your attention away from your illness. Take a class on stress-management. Learn relaxation techniques. Use every advantage you can to deal with stress: biofeedback, self-hypnosis, meditation. If you're ready, and here you'll need to check with your physician, go back to work part-time. The quicker you can get back into the mainstream of life, the quicker you'll recover.

How do I reduce stress?

Stress is your reaction to a given situation, not the situation itself. Thus, if you have learned to react by becoming stressed-out, you can also learn to react in a positive way.

Sometimes it is necessary to remove yourself from the situation. For example, you may no longer be able to handle your present occupation. You may have a need to change jobs. More often than not, however, it is a matter of learning to react differently to the same situation.

You may have to learn that you can't do everything at once, and that some things may have to wait until tomorrow. *What you also have to realize is that you can't take care of everyone's needs and take care of yourself at the same time. You must put yourself first.*

If you have physical limitations, explore the alternatives and don't focus on what you can't do. Finding new ways to react can be productive. Exercise will help relieve stress, as well. And so will the stress-reducing techniques mentioned in the previous questions. Remember, however, that these techniques only address the symptoms of stress and not the root causes. Those answers must come from inside you through an extensive examination of your activities, relationships and methods of relating. (See the section in Chapter Three on relieving stress.) The more control you have, the less stress you'll encounter.

Why do I feel so isolated?

Social isolation and a high degree of life stress increase the risk of death in cardiac patients four fold, according to the *New England Journal of Medicine*. For many patients of heart disease, the threat of death, whether real or perceived, creates a need to become self-reflective. This preoccupation may leave you feeling empty and alone, which may cause you to withdraw from people. To compensate, share your thoughts with a loved one or a health professional. This will diminish your sense of aloneness, and allow others to become part of your recovery program. But most importantly, it will give you a sense of "being connected" to someone else, which will greatly reduce your feelings of isolation.

Emotional sharing may be threatening and difficult to accomplish, especially for men. The risk of opening yourself emotionally creates thoughts of rejection, becoming enmeshed with another, loss of independence and perhaps loss of identity. However, the benefit of emotional sharing on a selective basis (such as with your wife, family or close friend) far outweighs the risk. It is also therapeutic and can increase your quality of life, an issue for most cardiac patients.

Can my mental state affect my physical state?

The mind and body are both part of a complex machine, with each dependent on the other. As a heart patient, you are naturally overly sensitive to your body's aches and pains, all of which may be referenced to your heart. As your mind continues to focus on these areas, you might notice that the pain increases. You may even feel a tightness in your chest and call your doctor. At the very least, you'll become frightened, which will increase the intensity of the pain.

Seemingly your pain is psychogenic, originating in your mind. But to be on the side of caution, check any and all pains with your physician. With time and healing you will find your body aches and pains less referenced to your heart, thereby requiring less attention. (The symptoms of a heart attack should always be checked out medically.)

Will my mental state be affected?

During a heart attack or during cardiac artery bypass grafting (CABG), the amount of oxygen received by the brain might be decreased for a brief period of time. The post-operative effects of this phenomenon are short-term memory loss, the inability to concentrate and confusion.

For most heart attack victims this condition is only temporary. It is a biochemical problem, in part, and nothing more. But for others less fortunate some degree of impairment may be permanent. In this case, you must learn to accept your condition and adjust your lifestyle accordingly. Explore your alternatives.

Why am I insecure?

Insecurity is the result of an inability to control your environment. You're unable to function without the help of medical personnel, your family and friends. You're uncertain about your health and future. You're afraid to overextend yourself, for fear of having another heart attack or further cardiovascular difficulties. These unknowns and many others contribute to your insecurity. *The more knowledge you have of a given situation, and the more you attempt to control that situation the more secure you're going to feel.*

Why do I feel so helpless?

The average person does not walk around thinking about heart disease. When it happens to you, you're shocked. "Why me?" you ask yourself. Strange faces tell you how to live your life. You're hooked up to equipment you've never seen before. When you leave the hospital, you feel as if you're leaving behind your life-support system. At home you may feel a need to cling to your wife, for fear that she will leave you because you are not the same person she married. All of this makes you feel dependent and helpless.

What you're feeling is valid and consistent with most, if not all, cardiac patients. What you will learn, in time, is how to manage your environment and reduce your fears and anxieties. As you rebuild your self-confidence, you will find a happy balance between what you can and cannot do.

FAMILY AFFAIRS

Why is everyone so nice to me? Am I going to die?

Everyone is nice to you because it's a natural reaction. Particularly your loved ones are just as confused and scared as you are. They want to be careful in how they treat you and what they say to you, for fear of exacerbating your condition. After all, they've been told that stress is bad for you.

But what they don't understand is that the more they overprotect you, the more stress and anxiety they create. You, on the other hand, think "If they're being so cautious around me then maybe they know something about my condition that I don't." It's important that your loved ones understand that you are not fragile and that you won't suffer a relapse if they treat you candidly. Let them know that you can handle the negative as well as the positive.

Will my condition affect my family?

The family unit is like a well-oiled machine. Each part is somehow dependent on the others in order for the machine to run smoothly. When a traumatic illness like heart disease strikes the family, everyone suffers. (*See* Chapter Four, Family Dynamics)

Early one Sunday morning in the spring of 1988, Bill (a former patient of mine) awakened his wife, Janet, and complained of severe chest pains — a crushing feeling, he told her, that made him feel nauseous. Janet rushed him to the emergency room of a Southern California hospital. A thousand images raced through her mind as the doctors examined Bill in the emergency room. "Is he going to die? What about the children? I can't believe this is happening."

11

Fortunately, Bill suffered only minimal heart damage from a moderate heart attack. But he and his wife, and their two children, learned the hard way how a life threatening illness can exacerbate existing conditions within the family unit.

Bill and Janet had been married 20 years, and to their friends it seemed like a happy union. But beyond their facade lurked a marriage in trouble. He was a bank executive who worked overtime at home in the evenings and on weekends to avoid facing his marital problems. As a result, their 8-year-old son, Rich, and their 10-year-old daughter, Chris, started having trouble in school.

After the heart attack, Bill became dependent on Janet. He also became irritable and depressed. Janet, on the other hand, came to resent the intrusion on her lifestyle, but she was afraid to confront Bill with her feelings for fear of aggravating his physical and emotional condition. This only caused more turmoil in their children's lives. Rich, who was too young to grasp the severity of his father's health problems, expressed his frustrations by fighting with schoolmates, while Chris started skipping school.

After months of counseling, Bill and Janet started to talk to each other about their frustrations and anxieties. They included their children in these discussions. Eventually, they became a much closer family then they had been prior to Bill's heart attack. Bill's priorities changed from an emphasis on work to an emphasis on family, and that brought the family closer together.

Bill and Janet's plight helps demonstrate that a *life threatening illness like heart disease doesn't have to destroy individuals within the family unit.* Placing your family before your job and learning to be open and honest with yourself and your family can create an emotional bond that will bring family members together.

CHAPTER TWO

SOUND MIND,
HEALTHY BODY

Heart disease is indiscriminate. It strikes both men and women, and it is the leading cause of death in the United States, responsible for 500,000 deaths per year. The emotional impact of heart disease is devastating for both victims and their families. In Chapter One we discussed the emotional trials and tribulations of this illness. We talked about the psychological impact it has on heart disease patients and how the family dynamics change because of a wide spectrum of emotional issues.

In Chapter Two we enter questions of a more general nature, but no less important. Full cardiac recovery requires both a sound mind and a healthy body. Although these answers are not intended for those seeking medical advice, they do help alleviate stress and anxieties related to certain misconceptions.

IMMEDIATE CONCERNS

Why did I suffer a heart attack?

People suffer heart attacks most often because of blocked coronary arteries. A myocardial infarction (otherwise known as a heart attack) occurs when the blood that flows to the heart is blocked. If the supply of blood is blocked for a matter of minutes, a portion of the heart muscle dies.

Coronary arteries become clogged because of a buildup of cholesterol, a waxy substance that circulates in the bloodstream. When too much cholesterol is produced or ingested, the arteries slowly become clogged. This condition is called atherosclerosis or hardening of the arteries. The American Heart Association estimates that more than 500,000 Americans die every year from this disease.

You can reduce the amount of cholesterol in your system and decrease your chances of heart disease by changing your diet. A 1984 study found that men who reduced their cholesterol cut their chances of a heart attack by 50 percent (although recent evidence suggests that perhaps the relationship between cholesterol and coronary heart disease is not quite as profound). Foods high in cholesterol include egg yolks, meat and high-fat dairy products. Of course, smoking, high blood pressure and diabetes are also contributing factors to coronary disease.

Others suffer what is known as a "silent heart attack." Roughly three to four million Americans fall into this category. Except for the lack of pain and non-existent symptoms, this type of heart attack is virtually the same as the more common variety, which is accompanied by pain and symptoms.

The only way to determine whether or not you've suffered a silent heart attack is with an electrocardiogram and/or stress treadmill. A previous "silent" heart attack makes you a likely candidate for a fatal heart attack.

Stress also contributes to heart disease. It is created when you perceive yourself as being unable to perform to a self-imposed level of expectation. Learn to recognize the physiological reactions to stress such as increased heart rate, higher blood pressure, sweating, feelings of confusion and an increased hormonal output like adrenalin, which increases your heart rate. If you have already suffered a serious heart attack, it would be wise to reduce your stress by making changes in your life. Classes on stress management can help you learn to relax and explore alternative reactions to stressful situations. All these responses will influence the way your body responds, thus decreasing your chances of serious cardiac disease.

What are my limitations?

Your physician is the only one qualified to answer this question. However, in most instances self-perception plays a key role in reaching beyond your so-called limitations. For example, heart disease patients often are afraid to have sex because they "perceive" the physical exertion as being too demanding for the heart.

The only way to relieve your fears is to ask your physician questions, or talk to him or her about entering a cardiac rehabilitation program. *The more control you have over your illness the less anxiety you'll experience. And knowledge is the beginning of self-control.*

With serious illness, "secondary gain" can also impede rehabilitation. Simply put, the benefit you derive from having someone take care of you only re-enforces your sick role. This pattern — which can become "habit-forming" — is a difficult one to break. The time to push yourself is after you have received the go-ahead from your doctor. Take baby steps at first. Walk up and down a flight of stairs before you walk around the block. If you feel any pain call your physician.

It's scary to push yourself beyond perceived limitations. In extreme cases, your fear can turn you into a psychological invalid — someone who is afraid to try anything. Although some dependency is necessary (i.e., medication and certain medical procedures that require a trained professional), do as much for yourself as you are physically and mentally capable of doing. This will increase your self-confidence and allow you to attempt more activities.

Why do I feel pain when there is nothing medically wrong?

The mind is a powerful tool. It can deceive you, and it can heal you. Some doctors have noticed that, following a heart attack, some patients seem to go into a decline which has little to do with the actual course of the disease. Here it may be your reaction to heart disease that is the causal factor. Research has shown how a patient's reaction to his or her illness can influence the ways in which the body responds.

"Phantom Pains" are the result of an oversensitivity to your illness. All aches and pains, no matter how small and insignificant, will typically be referenced to your heart. In fact, chest pains can become so severe they can feel as though you're actually suffering another cardiac event. It is this fear of another heart attack and the fear of having to undergo further surgery that triggers these feelings.

Just remember that this is an extremely common reaction for patients of heart attacks. In time — maybe three months to a year — your sensitivity to aches and pains will diminish, and the "chest pains" will become less frightening. (However, chest pains that last more than a couple of minutes should motivate you to seek medical help immediately.)

Why has my memory gone bad?

Cardiac patients often feel as though they're losing their minds because they can't remember where they placed their reading glasses or the name of a recent acquaintance. Frequently, this condition is the result of the heart-lung machine that was used during bypass surgery.

The brain requires blood and oxygen in order to function efficiently. One of the drawbacks of the heart-lung machine is that the brain sometimes doesn't receive enough oxygen. Heart attacks create a similar reaction. When this happens, you could well have short-term memory loss. Usually, this condition is only temporary. Only occasionally is it permanent or the recovery less than satisfactory. In this case adjustments will have to be made.

It is not uncommon for most cardiac patients to become preoccupied with their illness and loss of memory in its mildest form. It can confuse the best of us. Give yourself at least six months to a year to return to normal. Pace yourself, and don't expect too much in the beginning; adjust your plans and activities to compensate. You will experience less frustration this way.

ADJUSTMENTS TO MAKE

What is a Type A personality?

The people who possesses this type of personality are workaholics who push themselves too hard, almost to death — quite literally speaking. People like this find it hard to relax, and feel guilty when they do. They are impatient, although they come across as well-adjusted. Oftentimes, they are obsessive about success. Success to them may manifest itself in owning the most things; this materialism comes at the expense of their sense of inner being — a sense of being centered or grounded. An emotional "connection" is impossible for this person.

Should I enter a cardiac rehabilitation program?

Even if there are no physical reasons why you should enter a cardiac rehabilitation program, there certainly are impressive psychological benefits to be gained from such a program. Not only does it give you a sense of accomplishment, but it reassures you that your heart can withstand the physical exertion. Moreover, a rehabilitation program allows you to observe and participate with other patients with whom you can identify.

But a cardiac rehabilitation program can also create added anxiety. It's an unfamiliar environment that forces you to push yourself beyond your perceived limitations. It's up to you to let the staff know how you're feeling, especially if you're feeling dizzy or nauseous, or feeling any pain.

Some patients have been going to a cardiac rehabilitation program for years. It gives them a sense of security in knowing that professional help is available, and it gives them a support group to share their feelings. It also helps motivate them to continue to exercise. Many patients will not exercise on their own. Ask your doctor to prescribe a program, or at least discuss it with him or her.

Can I still maintain my quality of life?

Of course. Most of us have become used to a lifestyle that is not particularly healthy. We eat too much, exercise too little and, in general, don't take care of ourselves physically or emotionally.

Switching diets is a major readjustment, but not insurmountable. It requires that you become open to new tastes and smells, and that you become receptive to cooking with new spices that replace old habits like butter and salt. You can find these new spices in the market. And don't think "all or nothing," either. Think moderation. Eating an occasional piece of red meat or bowl of ice cream is okay — if it's done in moderation.

Learning to exercise may be a difficult task — because you're not used to working specific muscle groups — but as you begin to notice the physical and psychological changes, you'll feel better, look better and want to exercise more. The results you receive from cardiograms, stress treadmill tests, and blood samples may be good measures of your progress.

Although diet and exercise have an impact on your quality of life, certainly the way you relate to others and the way they relate to you will have the biggest impact on the degree of quality in your life. It is the sense of being emotionally connected with yourself and others that will increase your quality of life, more than anything else.

How do I regain control over my life?

You start by admitting to yourself that you are not a victim of heart disease, only an unwitting participant. Accept responsibility for your condition. If you put the blame elsewhere, you place the responsibility for change elsewhere. Educate yourself about your illness. Find out what you need to do in order to adjust your lifestyle. Welcome new information, whether from your body or from books. Ask questions of your doctor or nurse. Look at your illness from more than a single perspective.

Examine the cardiac risk factors in your life. Armed with this information you can better fight heart disease and deal with the changes. Don't wait for someone else to dictate your lifestyle. This will only create resistance. Make your own decisions. Begin to focus on the present and the future and away from your past. All of your resources (i.e., health professionals, family, friends) will give you the support you need to continue to be in control.

Will I always have to worry about what I eat?

Yes. The only healthy diet is one that is low in animal fat and cholesterol. You need to control your weight. Studies have shown a direct link between coronary heart disease and diet. Unfortunately, most heart disease patients are used to eating foods rich in cholesterol and other fats.

Cook without butter or oils, although some oils (mono and polyunsaturated) are said to help remove cholesterol from the system. Keep in mind, however, that they are still fats and should be used in moderation. Learn to acquire new tastes. Experiment with different recipes and spices. At first, the new diet may not seem like much fun, but if you share the grocery shopping and food preparation with your spouse, it could help create emotional closeness. At the very least, it could be fun and maybe even tasty.

INTERPERSONAL CONFLICTS

Is it okay to have sex?

Byron suffered a heart attack during the summer of 1989. Soon after he was released from the hospital, he started having sex with his wife on a regular basis. She became concerned because Byron was more amorous than he was prior to his heart attack. She felt as though he were trying to prove to himself and to her that he was still physically fit.

Phil, on the other hand, was afraid to exert himself sexually after his heart attack. He shied away from any physical contact with his wife because he feared that sex would require that he exert himself to the point of further cardiac complications.

Byron and Phil represent two approaches to resumed sexual activity. For the former it is excessive and for the latter it is too cautious. The healthy person falls somewhere between these two extremes. But for the cardiac patient, Byron and Phil present typical responses.

Certainly, one's desire for sex and the ability to perform may initially decrease because of a preoccupation with the illness. Thoughts of surgery and death may preclude your interest in anything as enjoyable as sexual activity. Anxiety, depression and blood pressure medication may also diminish sexual desire. But the healthy cardiac patient understands these limitations and frustrations and accepts new challenges by communicating with his or her partner.

Although you need to check with your physician first, in most instances sexual activity can be resumed after a brief period. In fact, some cardiologists believe that a cardiac patient can return to normal sexual activity as soon as he leaves the hospital. The psychological benefit of this activity may far outweigh the physical. In reality, sex requires no more energy than it takes to walk up two flights of stairs. But the emotional closeness created by sexual activity will, by its very nature, lessen the patient's sense of isolation, and create a bond with his partner.

Why doesn't the medical staff just tell me what to do?

Since each person's medical prognosis is different, therapy has to be refined for each individual program. Although it may

21

look as though each person is doing the same exercises, in fact, each is progressing at a different rate. Comparing yourself to others puts you at a disadvantage. Therefore, the responsibility for understanding your therapy and knowing your limitations falls on your shoulders.

Prepare a list of questions for the medical staff. They can't read your mind. This interaction will also allow you to become familiar with the rehab staff (one researcher found that patients who were unfamiliar with the medical staff were five times as likely to die suddenly). Push yourself in rehab. It's the only place where you'll have medical assistance and medical feedback of your progress. The staff is there to tailor a program to your needs. But they need your feedback, in exchange.

All I can think about is myself. Is this normal?

You've just had your world turned upside down. Your thoughts race from death to surgery and back to death again. Everyone around you has focused his or her attention on you. You're feeling dependent and needy. Selfishness, to the point of feeling insensitive to others (at this stage of the game), is a perfectly natural reaction. But as your condition improves, you should find yourself focusing less on your illness and more on your life with your family.

Howard and Nancy had been married for 20 years at the onset of his heart problems. He was an attorney who was very involved in his demanding law practice. Even so, he always found the time to be with his family. His two children adored him, and he and his wife experienced a freedom with each other that was rare.

Nancy's full time job of child-rearing and housekeeping kept her busy too, but she always made her husband and children a priority. The entire family had learned the key to a healthy relationship — emotional closeness.

Howard's heart attack came without warning and created a sense of panic for the entire family. Of course, Nancy and the two children, 13 and 15, were at his side as quickly as they could drive to the hospital. Groggy from medication and only slightly aware of his surroundings, Howard held Nancy's hand and fought for his life.

As the medical crises passed, Nancy and the kids began to experience an insensitivity in Howard that left them feeling frustrated and frightened. He seemed withdrawn and empty. Where there was once emotional warmth, there was now only a void. He had emotionally isolated himself from everyone.

Nancy spoke with Howard's physician about her concern and was relieved to know that such a reaction was not uncommon. The entire family was referred to someone who could help them understand the situation and address the issue.

As Howard began to understand the effect of his emotional isolation upon his family he was able to break through this "shell" and reach out to his family once again.

What is my wife's reaction to my condition?

Your wife has probably devoted herself to you since the heart attack. Her needs have been neglected. She may even feel as though you don't love her anymore. All she wants, really, is some justly deserved recognition and understanding. She needs to know that you still care for her, appreciate her and love her.

The emotional distress experienced by your spouse may be similar to your own — although for her, it may not present itself until three to 12 months post cardiac event. Indiscriminate crying, appetite and sleep disturbances and general emotional instability are the most common symptoms found among cardiac spouses.

It's imperative that you give her signs that you still love her. *Marriage does not stop with heart disease.* Talk to your spouse. Tell her that you care for her, but that your attention is elsewhere. Explain to her that she needn't be afraid to expose you to the negative for fear of worsening your condition. This is a misconception that produces emotional distance and anxiety.

Heart disease is extremely serious, but it's no excuse to isolate yourself from the rest of the world. Perhaps your spouse is just as frightened as you are. It is essential for you to reach out to those around you, especially now. Take the initiative.

Mary's husband had just suffered a massive heart attack where 30 percent of his heart muscle had been damaged. Naturally, he became self-absorbed and reflective. His lifestyle changed, and his attitude toward life changed. Mary became his caretaker, and he treated her as if she were a servant. Her life beyond his illness was nonexistent. She wondered if she had pushed her husband to the point of a heart attack.

After months of carrying around this emotional baggage, Mary's frustration level went off the charts. She resented her lifestyle, her husband's attitude toward her and the fact that she was taking care of him. But she swallowed these feelings for fear of exacerbating her husband's condition. Over time, she seriously considered divorce, but her commitment and devotion to her husband prevented any immediate action.

Eventually, Mary and her husband sought professional help. Once they understood the dynamics of heart disease and how it affected them emotionally, they were better equipped to deal with each other's frustrations and anxieties. Mary learned to relieve herself of the guilt she felt for her husband's illness, and her husband learned to better appreciate her feelings. Understanding your family dynamics will help lessen the need for self-absorption.

(Refer to Chapter Three, The Cardiac Spouse, and Chapter Four, for how a husband is affected by his wife's cardiac event.)

Should I seek counseling?

If you are feeling isolated and distant from friends and family, or if you are having difficulty adjusting to your changing lifestyle, eating habits, or new patterns, then professional guidance would be appropriate. You might want to go to your doctor or the rehab nurse for a referral. Find a therapist who has experience with heart disease. Check with your insurance company for coverage. At the very least, utilize your family and friends to help smooth the wrinkles to a healthier lifestyle.

Why can't cardiac rehab include a religious component?

It can. The spiritual component to cardiac rehabilitation is always available. Your family clergy person may well be able to meet your needs. For others, hospital clergy are available.

CHAPTER THREE

THE CARDIAC SPOUSE

The typical male cardiac patient turns first to his wife for emotional support. How she responds can have a direct impact on his recovery. (Please refer to end of chapter for a husband's role in his wife's recovery.)

GIVE ME STRENGTH

As the cardiac spouse, you must first help yourself by learning about the physical and emotional limitations of your husband's heart disease. As your knowledge in this area increases, the patient will become more confident in your ability to take care of him and yourself and you will understand more about what he experiences. As his caretaker, you may have to wear a number of hats: mother, wife, housekeeper, breadwinner. Keeping your wits about you will be challenging.

Any attempts to return to pre-illness roles too soon will only complicate the patient's recovery.

Further complicating matters will be the Delayed Reaction Syndrome. You may think you have everything under control. But three to 12 months down the road, after the patient is on the way to recovery, you may start feeling depressed, frustrated or angry. Look for telltale signs in yourself such as irritability, low frustration tolerance, sleep and eating disorders, a general sense of tiredness. You may need to seek professional help as these signs appear. At the very least, share these feelings with the patient. It will increase his sensitivity to your needs and set the stage for an emotional union.

Your needs are important too and must be addressed as they arise. The first step towards accomplishing this task is to be able to recognize them. The questions that follow are representative of your needs as the cardiac spouse.

How do I get past the fear of whether he's going to die?

The loss of a loved one is always devastating. And certainly this is a distinct possibility when faced with heart disease.

To get past the fear of whether he's going to die, you must learn to focus your attention on other areas of your life. Naturally, death is foremost in your mind after a cardiac event. It may cause you to feel lonely and depressed.

But as the patient's health improves and he begins to resume his normal activities, the chances of an untimely death become less distinct (although life with a cardiac patient, as with anyone, is never guaranteed).

As a cardiac spouse, however, you must also address the issue of abandonment. "How do I take care of myself if he should die?" I've actually worked with cardiac spouses who didn't know how to balance a check book. This kind of dependency only compounds your fear of abandonment.

Prepare for the worst. Learn to take care of yourself. *Don't let the fear of death cause you to withdraw from life.* You may be angry at your husband for putting you in this position. This is a natural reaction and one that will fade — along with the issue of death.

Will I be able to take care of my husband?

You will have a strong tendency to become overprotective of the cardiac patient. Naturally, you're concerned about his well-being. You want to be a part of his recovery process so you take control of his treatment.

The best way to help your husband is to allow him to take care of himself. Certainly, you need to be an important part of the treatment process, but don't baby him. Don't allow yourself to become his full-time caretaker.

Family involvement means love and support. These two gifts have a tremendous impact on a patient's recovery. But watch out for pitfalls. If he ignores his medical therapy, for example, you may have the urge to steer him in the "right" direction. Be careful that you don't relieve him of the responsibility for his own treatment. He may think of you as a nag. If he does, open lines of communication and talk about it. Avoid the temptation of doing too much, however. He must learn to do for himself.

Tom had double bypass surgery shortly after his 50th birthday. From the outset, he seemed to take it in stride. He did not experience any loss of self-confidence, or any of the usual emotional features that are characteristic of most cardiac patients. Prior to his surgery, he exercised religiously. As soon as he was medically cleared, he resumed this activity.

His wife, June, had a difficult time with his recovery. She became furious when he wouldn't stick to his diet or to the regime his doctor had prescribed. The issue for June centered around her need to take care of him. And if that meant "nagging" her husband into eating the right foods, so be it. She drove herself crazy for something over which she had little or no control.

Once June realized that the best way to help her husband was to allow him to help himself, life became much easier for both of them. She rightly communicated her concerns to him, and he responded positively. He changed his diet out of deference for her and because he was made aware of his dietary restrictions. She, on the other hand, no longer had to come across as the overly-concerned wife.

Why are my children hard to manage?

When a disaster strikes the family, your children sense the desperation and frustration of both parents. If these children are under the age of 10 or so, their parents typically leave them out of the crisis and subsequent recovery period. Consequently, they are left alone to deal with their own emotions and the guilt they often feel, believing it is somehow their fault.

The best way to handle this situation is to be open and direct with your children about the so-called disaster. Use simple language when defining the problem. Even if they don't ask, tell them about the heart attack and describe for them the emotional changes they are about to experience. The more they understand, the better. Keep it simple and let them know you love them and that they are not to blame. (*See also* Chapter 4, Children of Cardiac Couples)

Why am I angry?

Anger is one of least understood emotions, and the most difficult one to accept.

You are going through a rough period. Your role within the family has changed, leaving you confused and anxious. You may feel as though this change was forced upon you, thanks to your husband's heart attack. This is a normal reaction. After all, *look what he did to the family*. You now have to take care of him, the family, family business and other chores. He probably doesn't even notice your efforts, which makes you feel unappreciated, abused at times and unloved. As a professional, I would be more concerned if you didn't feel this way.

To overcome these feelings, you must address them before they become a problem. Talk about them with the cardiac rehab staff, your physician or clergyman. More importantly, talk to your husband. Communication will help to clarify the issues. Let him know how you feel about him, but do it in a productive, non-threatening way. In the long run, it will help both of you to understand each other just a little bit better, which will make the recovery process less stressful.

How do I deal with my husband's anger (and his denial of this anger)?

Most cardiac patients are angry and frustrated with the idea of losing a lifestyle to which they have become accustomed. Most cardiac spouses are afraid to be direct and honest with their husbands for fear of causing disharmony or further cardiac difficulty. By responding passively you are, in effect, encouraging his behavior. Cardiac patients need to learn to deal with situations that may be upsetting.

The first step to coping with your husband's anger may be to address the denial of his own hostility. Do so in a constructive manner by sharing with him your perceptions of the situation. Show him that you understand his need for denial. It will help lessen the pain. If he becomes defensive, tell him you'll come back later to discuss it when he's feeling less angry.

Right now he is feeling insecure and inadequate in many areas of his life. He's likely to respond defensively. Disarm him by letting him know that his illness has affected you, too. Tell him that you need to support each other through open and direct communication.

From a distance, Dave seemed calm and in control of himself — even after his cardiac difficulties. He followed the doctor's orders like a good soldier: he took his medicine, participated in cardiac rehabilitation and stuck to his new diet.

It wasn't long, however, before Dave — who was only in his late 30s — reverted back to his old ways of taking control of his life and everyone else's. Naturally, his wife became concerned.

This had been Dave's third heart attack in two years. One would have thought he had learned his lesson. Instead, with each heart attack he further suppressed his emotions. He was, in effect, a walking time bomb waiting to explode.

I witnessed first hand his anger one day in my office. After the usual round of questions, Dave became enraged for no apparent reason. He started yelling at his wife and at me, yet he could not admit his anger. When I pointed it out, he just turned a deaf ear. It took many more rounds of therapy before his wife and I were finally able to penetrate Dave's protective shield. Once we did, however, his anger became obvious; it didn't take long before Dave began to realize the connection between his emotional health and his physical health. This knowledge helped him on his road to recovery.

Why do I feel isolated and empty?

You probably feel abandoned by your husband. He has been taken away from you suddenly, and you're finding yourself in a rather precarious position. At first, your thoughts may be centered on his needs and away from your own. As you continue to ignore yourself, you are, in effect, isolating yourself from the world. That empty feeling in the pit of your stomach is telling you that you need that emotional connection again with your husband, or with others close to you.

Allow your husband and others to share selectively in your grief with all of its fear and confusion. Let them know about your feelings and your needs. In time, this empty, isolated feeling will go away.

Why aren't we handed more information in the beginning on the psychological aspects of heart disease?

At the time of the medical crisis, you and your family are preoccupied with your husband's physical well-being. The psychological issues don't usually come into play until after the medical emergency has passed. Typically, doctors will start talking about cardiac rehabilitation at this time, but may ignore the psychological issues of heart disease. Part of the problem is that many hospitals don't have enough trained personnel to accommodate this need, although referrals are common.

It is your responsibility to ask for this information and to seek out a qualified professional who can answer your questions. A good place to start is with your husband's cardiologist. Since I usually see the cardiac spouse three to six weeks post cardiac event, I suggest you seek information immediately after the medical crisis to avoid some of the early confusion and anxiety.

Should I confront my husband with my concerns, or is this just adding fuel to the fire?

Confront your spouse, but do it in a positive, productive manner, using the pronoun "I" to begin your statements, i.e., "I feel," "I need," "I want." This way your confrontation is clear and direct. Many cardiac patients are like children. They will test you. Cardiac patients, except in rare cases, are not fragile so don't treat them as if they were. Treat them as you would anyone else — with love and understanding.

WHAT'S GOING ON WITH THE PATIENT

My husband is much more affectionate since the heart attack. How do I relate to him in this new way?

Over the years, couples develop certain patterns of intimacy. When these patterns are interrupted with something as serious as heart disease, the relationship may suffer. If you were used to him as a non-expressive partner, and suddenly he's much more affectionate, it could cause complications.

Your husband just suffered a potentially lethal heart attack. This kind of crisis provides one with reason to reexamine thoughts on death and love. It is not uncommon to see a patient who was emotionally removed from his wife suddenly become warm and giving. This may make you feel as though you're being smothered. You need to explore this feeling and learn to recognize how it affects your ability to achieve and maintain a close relationship with your husband.

Learn new ways to relate to each other. This may require an adjustment period. Who knows? You may discover a new dimension to your relationship by opening yourself emotionally to him.

Why does my husband resent healthy people?

His resentment is not so much directed at healthy people but at himself for not having chosen a healthy lifestyle. Instead of berating himself, which creates emotional scars for both of you, he takes it out on others. For some patients, anger and resentment become debilitating. Therefore, it's important to expose these issues as quickly as possible.

Cardiac patients need to feel as if they're in control. Any sense of helplessness only leads to additional anger. He may also feel as though he was never given enough information about his illness and its effects, which creates additional anger, to be directed at others. Cardiac patients are preoccupied with their condition, making them insensitive and resentful of others. At times, these emotions may manifest themselves in anger. It is always more palatable to project these feelings on to others than to blame yourself. To do so, however, does not relieve the patient of the responsibility of these feelings, and at some point he will have to address these issues for himself — perhaps with your help.

Why won't he let me leave the house without him?

He probably feels as though you're going to abandon him. His only real sense of security is in knowing that his physician and his wife are still behind him and nearby. He may also be afraid that if something should ever happen to you, he would be left alone to deal with his life-threatening illness — and he's not sure he could handle that. This may cause problems when you want to leave the house for a few hours.

You need to take care of yourself. If leaving the house for a few hours is part of that program, then let him know. Tell him that you'll check up on him from time to time. Give him emergency numbers, in case they should become necessary.

Teach him how to take care of himself. *You do not have to give up your life to accommodate his insecurities. It is important for both of you to resume your normal activities as soon as possible.*

Why are we afraid to travel?

A serious cardiovascular event compels the victim and his family to "attach" themselves to a cardiologist. This person becomes the patient's lifeline by providing security. Travelling means leaving your cardiologist behind. For many patients and their families this fear is devastating, even though cardiologists can be found across the country and around the world.

Plan short trips, at first. As time goes on, you can lengthen these trips and the distance you travel. Prove to the patient that he can survive without his cardiologist — who, by the way, is only a phone call away.

FOR BETTER OR WORSE

He's pushing me away emotionally. What should I do?

One of two things usually happens when a coronary patient first comes home from the hospital. He will either withdraw into himself, or he will become needy and clingy. If he's pushing you away, it's because he's self-conscious and reflective. He's more focused on himself and his illness. He also may be trying to protect himself from any further emotional pain, although in reality his isolation is only increasing the pain.

I remember one patient who told me that he wanted to be as far away from his family as was humanly possible so that when he died his family wouldn't be distraught. Clearly, nothing could be further from the truth. Emotional distancing only leads to loneliness and bitterness.

One way to handle your husband's distance is to learn as much as you can about his emotional state. Talk with his cardiologist. Read books, such as those listed in the bibliography. Participate in his recovery program; be a part of what he has to learn so that you can learn too. You also may need to seek professional help in the form of a knowledgeable counselor to help bridge that emotional gap. One or two sessions may be all you need. Let him know that emotional isolation only increases his chances of a second heart attack. Perhaps this knowledge will motivate him to share.

Sex is a scary issue for me. What can I do about overcoming this fear?

It may help you to know that sex requires no more energy than it takes to walk up two flights of stairs. Only in extremely rare cases has any one ever died during sex, and the exact cause was never fully explained.

Your concern that your husband may over-exert himself is certainly understandable. Start out with less strenuous activities. The side-by-side (or spoon) position, for example, requires less exertion than any other position. Be creative. Explore new territory. Above all else, enjoy yourselves.

Why is my husband nice to others, but mean to me?

Try to understand your husband's frame of mind. He has just suffered a serious illness. He's angry at himself and at the world. You are his most convenient target, but it's not you he's really angry with. He's angry at his inability to take care of himself and his family. He wants his independence back, and he resents having someone take care of him, especially you.

He's fully aware of the fact that physical and emotional changes have taken place, and that he's turned into an angry person. Unfortunately, he doesn't know how to stop the anger.

When other people are around, he's more likely to bottle up his rage, which only adds to his frustration. Maybe he's not fully aware of how his actions affect you. Share with him how you have been impacted by his anger by telling him how it affects you, not by placing blame. Help him release his emotions in more productive ways by showing him the reasons for his anger and by letting him know that you want to help him and can act as a sounding board.

Why can't I stop mothering him?

Some of us use the role of caretaker to fulfill our own desires to feel wanted and needed. When there's a patient around who has a tremendous need to be cared for, a pattern of unhealthy dependency develops that's hard to break.

You and your husband may be feeding off each other's needs. You may be feeling anxious and afraid. He may be feeling helpless. Your inability to stop this "feeding frenzy" may be due, in part, to your husband's lack of desire to have the process stopped.

You must learn to trust your husband's abilities to do for himself (without harming himself, of course), and direct your desire to be wanted and needed towards those who can respond from a healthy position. Close friends and relatives may be just what you need right now.

How do I return to my previous role?

You must first decide whether you want to return to your previous role. If you do, you must be willing to give up the responsibilities of your new role. Many spouses find that they can no longer be happy with the old roles because their lives have actually become more interesting, with added responsibilities. Most change produces unexpected rewards, although it may be some time before these rewards are realized.

WHAT ABOUT ME?

Why am I lonely?

Ever since your husband's cardiac emergency, it appears as though the world's attention has focused on him. Doctors and nurses have taken care of his medical needs. Friends and relatives have stopped by for visits. Your children have treated him kindly. And you have sacrificed your world to take care of his needs. You feel abandoned and neglected.

You need to feel "connected" again to your husband and family. Knowledge, communication, understanding and empathy are the ways to accomplish this goal. Be realistic though, it may take awhile before your husband can respond to you in the way you need. Your family, however, has just as much of a need for emotional connection as you do. Take advantage of this situation and reduce your sense of loneliness by communication with them.

How can I think of myself when he's so sick?

Don't feel guilty about wanting to take care of your needs. There's more to your life than taking care of your husband. Take some time for yourself. Meet with friends, visit a relative, take in a movie. *Do whatever it takes to regenerate yourself. It will help relieve some of the stress in your life, and give you the energy necessary to help take care of him.*

Why do I feel abused and unloved?

Your husband is preoccupied with his condition. He believes everyone and everything exists solely for his recovery. He expects you to do as much as possible to ease his suffering, and since you probably do more than you need to, you feel abused and unloved. He doesn't realize that there are limits to how far he can push you. He probably hasn't taken the time to thank you for your efforts or even thought of doing so. And if you haven't confronted him by saying "I am feeling abused and unloved," or "I need to know that you love me," you have only yourself to blame.

The more you neglect your own needs, the more you are going to resent your husband. Don't isolate yourself either. It will help diffuse the overwhelming sense of emotional closeness you need from you husband.

When do *my* needs get met?

The sooner you learn that your husband can do for himself, the sooner your needs will be met. But you must give your husband room to prove himself. He must learn what his limitations are and how far he can push the boundaries. In time, he will rebuild his self-confidence and self-esteem.

Although you may feel guilty about leaving him on his own, it is a necessary step to full cardiac recovery. He must learn to separate himself from his caretaker — you. This will free up your time and allow you to meet your needs without guilt.

How do I help my spouse relieve the stress in his life?

Your mate is the only one who can change his or her life situation. You can help, however, by exploring those areas which may be creating stress. As you do so, you might examine these areas for yourself as well, and then you can both share the information with each other. This interchange in and of itself will help to reduce stress and create emotional closeness. Typically stress inducers are found within the work environment and/or from personal life events. What follows is a detailed examination of both of these areas. Check what is appropriate for each of you and discuss it with your mate.

Four areas of your spouse's job that may be causing stress:

1) Work overload
2) Occupational environment
3) Work relationships
4) Personal and general concerns

Seven areas of personal life that may be causing stress:

1) Personal relationships
2) Home environment
3) Leisure activities
4) Quality time with family
5) Personal time
6) Financial concerns
7) Cardiac illness and recovery

Use the following charts (Table A for job, Table B for personal life) to help better define the stress in your spouse's life, then examine the alternatives and formulate a plan of attack.

Table A

1) WORK OVERLOAD

_____ Has trouble finishing work on time
_____ There are too many interruptions
_____ There are not enough work breaks
_____ Work schedule is inflexible
_____ Expected to work too many hours
_____ Inundated with too much paperwork
_____ Has too much responsibility
_____ Work is not satisfying
_____ Work is not consistent with training and
     education

2) OCCUPATIONAL ENVIRONMENT

_____ Has an insufficient amount of work space
_____ The noise level is intolerable
_____ The lighting causes headaches
_____ Management is unresponsive
_____ No room for professional growth
_____ Policies and procedures are too stringent
_____ Feeling as though stagnating at work
_____ Company has a high turn-over rate
_____ Receives poor employee benefits
_____ Has no time for training classes
_____ Doesn't have proper supplies and equipment

3) WORK RELATIONSHIPS

_____ Has conflicts with peers
_____ Has conflicts with supervisors
_____ Has conflicts with management

WORK RELATIONSHIPS *continued*

_____ Management doesn't respect him/her
_____ Peers don't respect him/her
_____ Supervisors don't respect him/her
_____ Has no authority
_____ Doesn't receive deserved recognition
_____ Lack of performance feedback
_____ Lack of cooperation among employees
_____ Team effort goes unrewarded

4) PERSONAL AND GENERAL CONCERNS

_____ Professional recognition
_____ Inadequate training to do job effectively
_____ Expectations are inconsistent with the
 realities of job
_____ He/she is a workaholic
_____ Salary is not commensurate with training
_____ Professional values and organization values clash
_____ Personal problems affect job performance

Table B

1) PERSONAL RELATIONSHIPS

_____ Lacks honesty
_____ We have a hard time communicating
_____ Our sex life is in trouble
_____ One of us is manipulative
_____ One of us verbally abuses the other
_____ One of us is physically abused
_____ There is no closeness in our relationship

2) HOME ENVIRONMENT

_____ Our home is uncomfortable
_____ Our home is too crowded
_____ The noise level in our home is too high
_____ Our home is unattractive

3) LEISURE ACTIVITIES

_____ Leisure activities leave him/her unsatisfied
_____ Prefers to be alone

4) QUALITY TIME WITH FAMILY

_____ Communication is superficial
_____ We spend little time together as a family
_____ There's a lack of trust within the family unit
_____ Lack of emotional sharing within the family unit

5) PERSONAL TIME

_____ Doesn't get to spend enough time by himself/herself
_____ Doesn't like to spend time by himself/herself
_____ Wants to spend time alone, but doesn't know what to do

6) FINANCIAL CONCERNS

_____ We're experiencing financial difficulties

7) CARDIAC ILLNESS AND RECOVERY

_____ Has too many restrictions and limitations
_____ Illness has created family problems
_____ Medicine is causing side effects
_____ In conflict with the medical staff
_____ In conflict with the rehab staff
_____ Having emotional problems
_____ Having physical problems

Stress reduction is not just learning how to respond differently to those situations which are stressful to you. It has to be a combined effort that begins with an awareness of your stress factors. With this accomplished, proper nutrition and a consistent exercise program combined with healthy communication help to reduce life's stress by addressing their sources. Relaxation techniques such as deep breathing, muscle relaxation, guided imagery, self-hypnosis and biofeedback are useful but only address the symptoms of your stress, not the causes. An overall program which includes all or most of the above is necessary to effectively reduce your stress.

A HUSBAND'S ROLE IN HIS WIFE'S RECOVERY

Although women account for only 17% of all cardiovascular diseases annually, the issues they and their husbands must deal with during the recovery period are no less complicated. While the above needs and reactions of male cardiac patients are equally applicable to women, women may feel additional anxiety over the welfare of their families and their inability to provide the same care for their husbands. They may also be especially sensitive to their appearance after the heart attack, and exhibit concern that they are no longer attractive because of surgical scarring.

As the husband of a female cardiac patient, you must address these issues. She needs your assurances of your continued attraction and love. (Refer to Chapter Four for a focus on the special family concerns of the female cardiac patient.)

Will he still love me like this?

Cosmetic concerns because of heart bypass grafting manifest differently for men and women. It has been my experience that female patients have more concern about appearing young, soft and unblemished. Surgical scarring may present a problem to those who fall prey to this kind of thinking. The scarring may also create concerns over emotional issues related to sexual intimacy. I've had patients who refused to allow their mates to view or touch the scarred areas of the body.

Regardless of your gender, it is vitally important to address your concerns by sharing with your partner. This is the only person who can help you attain emotional intimacy which, in turn, will help you to return to "normal" activities as quickly as possible.

Diane was a 58-year-old woman who led an active life as a wife, mother, and a business manager of a large law firm. Her husband was a successful entrepreneur. He relied heavily on her to take care of the household duties, as well as their social life.

After her first heart attack, Diane lost energy and motivation. She became extremely depressed. Although it wasn't necessary for her to bring in the extra income, she felt it was her duty. When she could no longer work, her self-esteem suffered. She wasn't even sure she'd be able to take care of her husband and children, anymore.

When she looked in the mirror, and noticed her post-surgical scars and emaciated body, she wondered if her husband would still find her attractive. Her self-confidence was shattered.

Diane spent six months in therapy. Most of her treatment revolved around her husband. She tried to share with him her insecurities. Once she overcame that hurdle, the rest sort of fell into place. Her husband explained to her that he still loved her, and that he still desired her. Slowly, they were able to bridge the emotional gap that had prevented sexual intimacy.

CHAPTER FOUR

FAMILY DYNAMICS

It should be quite evident from your reading thus far that heart disease affects the entire family — from the oldest to the last born. No one is unaffected by this life-threatening illness. But only recently has the medical community acknowledged these changes.

One exception which, surprisingly, dates back to the 1940s, is *Patients Have Families* by Henry B. Richardson. Richardson was a man ahead of his time. He argued quite simply that patients should not be treated separately from their families.

Four Types of Family Interaction

Salvador Manuchin, a leader in the field of family therapy, characterized four types of interactions among family members who have been affected by chronic illness:

1) Enmeshment — Family members are overreacting to the stress of another member and demonstrating a lack of autonomy;
2) Overprotectiveness — The family members are not being allowed to handle their own problems;
3) Conflict Avoidance — Open airing of disagreement is not permitted and problems are not resolved;
4) Rigidity — Transactional patterns are repeated inflexibly, and change is resisted.

While all of these traits can be found in the cardiac family, the last three are almost always present.

Overprotectiveness, for example, comes about because of the wife's need to comfort her husband. She is afraid for him. She doesn't want him to exert himself to the point of further complications so she tries to do everything for him. If she has low self-esteem to begin with her need to overprotect her husband becomes even greater.

Typically in this kind of relationship, disagreements are avoided because the wife fears she may upset the patient (this is called Conflict Avoidance). She, in turn, takes on the role of peacemaker and pays a high price for this honor in terms of her own emotional and physical well-being. As the patient's condition improves, he gradually pulls away from his wife to regain his independence. Along the way he finds that she's resisting this change.

Roles are constantly being defined and redefined during a cardiac recovery. Rigidity makes it difficult to change. Open and direct communication among family members will help foster a healthy environment in which each participant is willing to change. Moreover, a clear understanding of each member's role within the family unit will become more important as change takes place.

Once these new roles have been firmly established, this new pattern of interaction begins to feel quite "normal," even if it seems unnatural. If these issues are left unattended, further problems can and will impede rehabilitation.

At the beginning of this book I tried to help you understand the impact heart disease had on my family. It was a painful experience for me to come to certain realizations about my family and myself. But at the same time it was a necessary evil because it helped create a pattern of communication that, in turn, helped pull us through my father's recovery period.

Diagram Techniques

One technique for learning about the way your family interacts is to have each family member draw a diagram, and then to sit down and compare them. Relationships between family members change as a result of a crisis such as a heart attack. It is worthwhile working through the process of drawing the diagrams, and then sharing them with your family. This exercise will illustrate more clearly how the family dynamics have changed — you can see it in front of you in black and white.

Start with a circle which represents your perception of how your family members relate to each other. Family members may be placed in or around the circle depending on how you relate to them. Draw lines between the different members of your family, using one line for a weak bond and two for a strong bond. The size of each person that you draw may also have meaning for you. For example, dominant people in the family might be drawn larger than the other members of the family; or emotionally weak persons (as you perceive them) might be drawn smaller than other family members. You might also find the need to draw more than one circle to represent your current family and your family of origin, for example your families before and after marriage.

You may draw or write about the people, places and things that have influenced your life. Some of you may have had a stronger bond with someone outside your family and you may want to indicate this bond with a line drawn between that person and yourself. (You can also be innovative and show this connection any way you wish.)

Expectations and feelings of yourself and of others in the family are an important part of behavior and should be written outside your circle in order for you to have a better understanding of what motivates your interactions. The diagram you draw is first a tool to make you aware of yourself within the family. It must then be shared with your family members to communicate how you are feeling and your perceptions of the family unit, and help you to understand their point of view. The communication that will arise between you and your family members in discussing what you drew will bring all of you closer together.

When discussing your diagram with your family, do it from your own perspective, from an "I" position (What I feel, What I see, What I need), rather than in an accusatory manner. Take time to listen to other family member's perspectives.

There is no right or wrong way to draw these diagrams. The process of communication that will result from discussion is what is important. You may find it useful to repeat this process as you progress in your cardiac recovery.

The following diagram is drawn from my perspective as an adult child of a victim of heart disease, showing my perceptions of my family life after my father's heart attack.

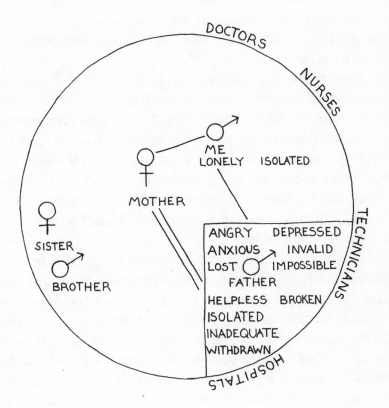

Inside the circle I have placed my mother, my father, my sister, brother and myself. Of note is the weak bond between my father and myself, represented by the single line. His heart attack in many ways only exacerbated already existing problems within our family. He had always been emotionally distant, and had been frequently absent from the family on business related trips. Notice the emotions that were characteristic of my father after the attack; the impact of these emotions was to wall him off even more from the rest of the family. Nonetheless, he remained the dominant person in the family as his illness dominated our family life.

My mother is the central figure because everything revolved around her. She was the placater, the mediator for the entire family. My brother and sister are drawn toward the outside of the circle because they are away at school, and seemed to me to be far removed from my life.

Even before the heart attack, I had feelings of loneliness, isolation and emptiness, and a strong codependency between my mother and myself already existed. My father's heart problems magnified these things. Any amateur psychologist could tell from the diagram that I was a loner during my childhood. I was either smothered by my mother or ignored by her because of my father's needs. To survive, I withdrew into my own little world. Naturally, this had a tremendous impact on my life and my future relationships.

Notice the absence of friends outside my circle. I never had friends and relatives because it was necessary to maintain quiet around the house during my father's recovery period, and relatives focussed on their own needs rather than of those of my family. Things that were once important to me, such as school, music, teachers and the boat we owned at the time — something which brought us together as a family in a way communication did not — were replaced by other important people and things. These consisted mostly of medical professionals who were present because of my fathers's illness.

Look at your own diagram. What do you see? What don't you see?

What is frightening to me about my diagram is that it shows the similarities between my father and myself. We both built up walls of isolation, and our lives were devoid of outside stimuli with the exception of the medical professionals. I found it difficult to relate to anyone or anything, explaining the lack of people, places and things outside my sphere. My mother remained the central figure in our lives as we competed for her attention. For obvious reasons, she focused on my father and his illness.

The medical professionals became a substitute for my family. Years ago it was all too common for families to have an extended family — children and grandparents and grandchildren all living under one roof. When illness struck, they helped each other during the recovery period by providing love and emotional support.

During the 1960s, 1970s and most of the 1980s, this country witnessed a shift from this type of family existence to one that was more independent. Family members became scattered across the country and abroad. When illness struck, "professional caretakers" were needed. These relationships were devoid of any real emotional closeness, which impeded recovery. Today, perhaps for economic reasons, "extended families" are coming back into vogue, and they're providing a partial answer to the health care problems of this country.

Self-Perception

Self-perception is the way in which you see yourself. You may see yourself as an assertive person in one situation, and as withdrawn in another. In either case, your self-perception will be a major factor in determining your behavior. For example, during my developmental years, my sister always related to me as the "younger brother" (she was 11 years older). In latter years, it was difficult for me to relate to her as an adult, because I still perceived myself as that young child.

In cardiac families, especially right after the medical crisis, the patient typically will see himself as being helpless and dependent (in its extreme form, this is known as psychological invalidism). As others begin to take care of him, his self-perception as a helpless dependent is reinforced. It's imperative for the patient to do as much for himself as possible, so as to build confidence and self-esteem from the outset of recovery.

Expectations: Overt and Covert

Expectations of yourself and those you have of others are one of the driving forces behind your behavior. *Overt* expectations leave little room for error. As such, everyone knows where they stand, even though they know their expectations may not be met. Conversely, *covert* expectations can lead to misunderstanding and create considerable conflict. With heart disease, the latter is more characteristic. In an attempt to avoid conflict, direct messages are avoided. Thus, covert messages produce the opposite of what is intended. These misleading messages may also provide the impetus to push oneself to a point of destruction.

WIFE

> *Honey, did I tell you that the family down the street just bought a new car. It's really nice. They also got their house painted.*

HUSBAND

> *Good for them. They can afford it. We can't.*

WIFE

> *I know. I just thought you'd want to know.*

The implied message here is one of despair over not being able to afford what her neighbors can afford. Her approach may leave her husband bitter and feeling as if he should provide more and push himself harder. Here's another example:

HUSBAND
> *I sure enjoyed dinner last night at the Frank's house. Ever notice how their place is always clean and organized. And the meals she prepares are incredible.*

WIFE
> *It was fun. She's quite a woman. I wonder why they don't have any children, though?*

HUSBAND
> *I don't know.*

The husband is sending his wife a covert message that says, "Why don't you keep house the way she does?" The wife volleys with another covert message about the fact that because the Franks don't have any children, it's easier for Mrs. Frank to maintain and organize the household.

Since heart disease changes family roles on an ongoing basis, expectations will be in a state of constant change, as well.

Ned was only 51 years old when he suffered his first massive heart attack. At the time, he had a high-level corporate job in the medical industry. The daily pressures of his job forced him to work overtime. The added stress in his life, along with his naturally aggressive personality, contributed to his illness.

His wife, Jeri, spent most of her time as a volunteer with a community welfare organization. She also took care of their three teenage sons. The oldest son, Mark, had just started college, while the other two were still in high school.

Ned had always been controlling with his wife and children. It was difficult for him to express his emotions. When he was home, his sons usually went off with friends, while Jeri kept to herself. They had developed a relationship that allowed everyone plenty of breathing room. Open displays of affection were rare.

Ned's heart attack forced a number of changes within the family unit. To begin with, Jeri, who never had to worry about their financial status, panicked when faced with the prospect of having to go out and earn money. She became childlike and unresponsive. The older son Mark was forced to take on the responsibilities of his father. Fortunately, he handled the situation well.

Within four months it became quite clear that Ned's condition would remain serious enough to warrant major changes in his work schedule. Although his savings were substantial, retirement would create hardship. Their lifestyle would be curtailed and their expectations altered. Ned would no longer be the family's dogmatic leader, which left Jeri and the three boys in a rather precarious position.

Jeri's image of her husband as the strength of the family had been shattered. She transferred these feelings to Mark, who remained at home instead of going back to college. Although it was a difficult transition for everyone, Mark took over the role of family provider until Ned was able to resume his role at the head of the table.

Ned's family provides an excellent example of changing expectations. Many cardiac families go through painful transitions during this period. The more you know about family dynamics, the more able you will be to communicate openly and directly with each other.

Dialogue

Throughout this book I often suggest counseling for those people who find it difficult to express their true emotions.

During the sessions I've held, I often give my counselees examples of how they can better communicate with their partners and/or family members. More often than not, I give them snippets of dialogue to encourage the process. This way there is no misunderstanding.

Here's an exchange between family members. Notice how they resolve their differences through open and direct communication.

HUSBAND
> *Lately I've been walking around in a daze.*

WIFE
> *How do you mean?*

HUSBAND
> *I feel lost, confused. I don't know what's going to happen to my life or to us.*

WIFE
> *I feel the same way, but to a lesser degree, I'm sure. Why do you feel that way?*

HUSBAND
> *I don't know. Maybe it's because there's so much I don't know about my health and the future. I'm scared.*

DAUGHTER
> *I'm scared, too.*

WIFE
> *I think we're all scared. But your daddy and I love you very much and we're going to work together.*

DAUGHTER
> *Are you going to die, daddy?*

HUSBAND
> *I don't think so, honey. At least, that's what the doctors tell me. But don't be afraid to come talk to me or your mother about it. Okay?*

WIFE
> *What else is bothering you?*

HUSBAND
> *I don't have any answers.*

WIFE
> *Me neither. But I think we need to take it one step at a time and keep talking to each other.*

This type of exchange reflects a family whose members are not afraid to communicate their feelings. They also don't blame each other or criticize each other. They comfort and nurture one another, which helps alleviate their pain.

Anger is one of the most prevalent emotions in cardiac patients and one of the more difficult to address. (Refer to Chapter 1, Why am I angry?) Here's an exchange between husband and wife in which the anger is slowly released.

HUSBAND
> *I wish you wouldn't make so much noise in the kitchen when I'm trying to rest.*

WIFE
> *I'm sorry.*

HUSBAND

> *I'd also appreciate it if you tell the kids to*
> *stop running around the house like a pack of wolves.*
> *Isn't it their bedtime, anyway?*

WIFE

> *Honey, why don't you just relax. Read a book or*
> *something. You're getting upset over nothing.*

HUSBAND

> *What do you mean, nothing? I'm not feeling well, and*
> *these outside irritations are causing pains in my*
> *chest. Why can't you be a little more understanding?*

WIFE

> *Why do you have to yell at me? I'm not the enemy,*
> *you know. Talk to me, I'm your wife. I love you and*
> *you're upsetting me. I know you're angry, so let's*
> *talk about it.*

HUSBAND

> *I've never been good at talking about my feelings.*

WIFE

> *I know, and I don't want to make you uncomfortable.*
> *But you've got to learn to talk about things instead*
> *of bottling them up inside you. You're making it*
> *harder on me and yourself. We're growing apart and*
> *that hurts me. Please, honey, let's talk about this.*

HUSBAND

> *I'm afraid. I know this is hard on you and I want*
> *to protect you from my pain and suffering.*

WIFE

But can't you see that by not sharing your feelings with me I feel left out, and that's tearing us apart?

HUSBAND

I'm sorry. It's just that I've been frustrated and I don't know how to handle it. My memory is not what it used to be, and that scares me. I realize I'm being hard on you and the kids, but sometimes I can't control myself. It feels like I'm going to explode. I just want everything to be the way it was before my heart attack.

WIFE

It's frustrating for me, too, you know. It hurts me to see you suffer like this. I want to help you, but I don't know how. But I think this is a good start. I think we need to talk about these issues and others. It helps me better understand what you're going through, and I think it's good for you, too.

HUSBAND

You're right. But I'm still afraid.

WIFE

Me too. That's why I think it's important that we lean on each other. We're a team.

Once the patient begins to release suppressed emotions, he finds it easier to deal with the recovery period of his illness. Obviously, both partners need to encourage each other to share openly and directly.

PLAYING A ROLE

The following questions and answer provide information to help clear some of the confusion surrounding family issues during recovery.

Will our family ever feel 'normal' again?

All families tend to develop specific patterns of interaction. Within these patterns are well-defined roles. Each member is "assigned" a role. He becomes, in effect, what others expect him to be. As long as these expectations are consistent with his self-image, everything is in order. Problems arise when there's a conflict.

With cardiac families, almost everyone will have to change not only their own role within the family unit, but their expectations of each other. Some family members may not be comfortable with these changes. It just doesn't feel normal. But as the new roles and expectations become more familiar, the old roles will become faint and a new sense of "normality" will begin to appear. Communication, however, is the key to a smooth transition.

DAUGHTER
> *Since daddy got sick, it's been really weird around here. Daddy and I don't joke around anymore, and that scares me. Did I do anything wrong? Is everything going to be all right?*

WIFE
> *We're all going through a lot of changes, dear. Especially daddy. He is having a difficult time dealing with his heart attack. But he still loves you very much. It's just that he's worried about his health.*

HEART TO HEART

HUSBAND

> You both mean more to me than anything else in the world. But I'm having a difficult time right now and it's hard for me to talk about it. I know there have been a lot of changes in this family, and that scares me.

WIFE

> What are you afraid of?

HUSBAND

> I'd rather not talk about it right now. It's too difficult.

WIFE

> Can't you see how frightened we are? We need to talk about this so we can help each other.

DAUGHTER

> I love you daddy. I want you to be better.

HUSBAND

> Okay. I'll try to explain this — I'm afraid that I won't be able to work again and to continue providing for this family. It worries me when I think about how all this will affect the two of you. I feel responsible, and that tears me apart.

WIFE

> I want to fix everything for you, and we both want to take care of you — but we don't know how. Tell us how we can help.

HUSBAND

> This isn't easy, but I need to know that you're not going to leave me.

WIFE

> *Leave you! Why on God's earth would we want to leave you? We love you.*

Will the chaos in our family affect the patient's health?

Cardiac patients typically exhibit low frustration tolerance. Noises and other minor disturbances will have an impact on his mood. No matter how this frustration manifests itself, it will have an impact on other family members. If he's the type of person who vents his frustration through expressions of anger, then the family will certainly bear the brunt of his outbursts. Activities for children such as listening to loud music or roughhousing with friends may have to be curtailed or carried out elsewhere. These irritations create added confusion and anxiety for the patient. Add to this the chaos and confusion present because of the many unknowns and fears associated with heart disease, and you have a situation in which hormonal increases could be cause for concern.

How do we know if our 'new' expectations of each other are realistic?

The *American Heritage Dictionary* defines an expectation as something that is reasonable, due, likely or certain. In families, repetitive behavior and attitudes set the stage for certain expectations. You may come to learn what is expected of others based on what they have produced in the past. When a medical crisis like heart disease occurs, it interrupts a family's routine. All former expectations are disrupted.

For the first few months, the patient's changing physical and emotional condition will dictate expectations. Once you become more aware of the patient's emotional and behavioral changes, you'll slowly start to build a new set of expectations. Give this process time to develop. Expectations which have a probability of being realized are realistic.

Remember that as roles change, so do expectations. Talk to each other about these changes. Express yourself.

I like my new role in life. But my husband, who is struggling to regain his authoritative position within the family, wants me to go back to my old role. How do we resolve this issue?

Your husband is used to behaving in a certain way when it comes to family matters. Until his cardiac difficulties, you may have been resigned to a specific family role. As his health improves, he will want the situation at home to return to his perception of "normal." But your concept of "normal" has changed.

He no doubt perceives the return of his role to the head of the household as a positive step toward full recovery. If he thinks you're trying to arm wrestle him for position, it would create considerable hurt and anger.

Communicate your differences. Sure, there may be some anger, resentment and frustration, but you need to clear the air about real and perceived changes. You need to negotiate a compromise that will leave both of you with some sense of victory. Healthy relationships require compromise, and compromise is the key to change. Communication is the tool that will make this work.

Why can't my family be more loving and giving?

In order for members of your family to become more loving and giving, they need to have security in the knowledge that they won't be rejected for sharing their feelings. Unfortunately, with heart disease, issues of abandonment may be overwhelming. The challenge, then, is to build secure relationship based on mutual trust and respect.

You must allow each member his or her feelings with regard to the changing roles within the family unit. You have to let them know it's okay to feel depressed or angry. Encourage them to express these feelings in productive ways. Build an environment in which everyone has an opportunity to share their emotions. In time, perhaps even as long as years, emotional sharing will become part of your daily lives. Don't give up. Be patient.

TRIALS AND TRIBULATIONS

Why do all of our problems seem so much worse since the heart attack?

Immediately after the heart attack, minor problems and irritations may seem greater because your energy is focused on the medical crisis. Consequently, everything else gets shelved.

Attend to these issues as soon as you can so that they don't become overwhelming. Sometimes, only a phone call is needed to solve something. Take it one step at a time.

When my husband gets angry, I fall apart and our children become unruly. How do I overcome these obstacles?

To better understand his anger, refer to Chapter One. You and your children must first understand the reasons for your reactions to his anger. You are acting out of fear, perhaps for your own safety. Learn to be more patient. You also don't have to treat your husband with kid gloves. Let him know how his anger is affecting you and the children. Sit down and talk to him about this. Do not allow yourself or the children to be emotionally abused.

My wife and daughter had a difficult time with my surgery. They're still worried that I may die. How can I help them overcome this fear?

Information and communication are the best weapons. The more information they have about heart disease and your particular condition, the better equipped they are to handle their concerns. This information must come from you or your doctor. Once all the information has been assimilated, sit down with one another and talk about your concerns and feelings. It's the best medicine for any emotional difficulties, and it provides a foundation for healthy relationships. With time and emotional intimacy, thoughts of death will become more infrequent.

THE FEMALE CARDIAC PATIENT

The issues for male cardiac patients have been examined quite carefully in the appropriate chapters in this book. Women account for only 17% of all cardiovascular diseases annually; nonetheless, recovery is just as difficult for them as for men.

Do family dynamics change when the patient is a woman?

The effect of heart disease on family dynamics with female patients is the same as with male patients: each family member is affected in one way or another. But the impact these emotions have on the patient may vary between the sexes, according to the amount of "emotional baggage" that has been built up over the years. Certainly, female patients are more likely to be aware of and express their emotions sooner than male patients. But both suffer equally.

Economic issues may also separate the sexes — if there is only one salary to depend on, and it happens to be that of the patient. For double-income families, the economic issues may be just as pressing. Abandonment looms large for both, and must be dealt with in short time in order to lessen the degree of anxiety.

The bottom line is the same for both sexes. No matter what the issues, emotional openness and directness is the only way each family member will feel a part of the recovery process as well as experience the necessary "emotional connectedness" necessary for healthy relationships.

How will they get along without me?

Female patients, although affected by the same emotional instability, experience additional anxiety over familial and caretaking concerns, such as "Who will take care of my house and my husband" and "How will he manage without me?"

The likelihood of the presence of young children in the home is slim, since 136,000 heart attacks per year occur within the 45-64 age bracket. Only 3,000 a year occur within the 29-44 age bracket. Thus, it is more likely that older teenagers and adult children will be present, either living at home or on their own. For the former group, although they may feel they can function independently, some supervision and structure is needed. For women the inability to meet this need only adds to the existing sense of inadequacy felt by most cardiac patients. Many of the female cardiac patients I have spoken with believed they could resume their normal household function immediately after returning home. The realization that this was not possible created added frustration which would manifest itself, typically, in irritable behavior. Of course, everyone in the family suffered the consequences.

Emotionally destructive consequences of heart disease can be minimized by addressing needs as they arise. For example, a professional housekeeper can be retained for as long as needed during the recovery process. If finances become a problem, certainly older teenagers can take on part-time work in order to help out. This will help them feel as if they are a part of their mother's recovery and perhaps create cohesiveness which lends itself to emotional closeness.

FOR CHILDREN OF CARDIAC COUPLES

Family roles change almost immediately after a heart attack, and children may take on parental roles as parents regress. When the patient is male, the female spouse may take on the role of primary (perhaps the only) wage earner while the patient is disabled. Children may take on caretaking duties of the patient as these new roles upset what Virginia Satere called family homeostasis (balance). A struggle to create a new balance will ensue, leaving family members with some sense of feeling uncomfortable and insecure.

To accommodate such feelings and dynamics, it is imperative for all family members, including the patient, to communicate to each other in an open, direct manner. In this way, everyone understands each other's emotions and how these emotions affect the entire family. Communication also allows each person to be aware of personal and family needs, thus allowing everyone to be included in the recovery process.

Older and/or married children of cardiac patients create additional dynamics. Facing one's own mortality becomes a pressing issue because of the fear and apprehension that manifests and eventually mandates a different style of life. Being married with children creates a conflict between your present family and your original family. How much time and energy can be focussed on the latter, without feeling guilty and neglectful of your own family? How can you not devote your time and energy to your parents who are now in need of your help? Creating a balance will be difficult at best, and at the very least create stress within your own family and a considerable amount of anxiety for you. Sacrifices such as nursing the sick parent (and spouse as well) or providing financial support may be necessary. You may even have to postpone educational or vocational plans in order to function as caretaker. It has been my experience that many adult children of cardiac patients take it upon themselves to do more than is really necessary, thereby creating unnecessary hardships for themselves and their family.

Don't attempt to take on the complete responsibility for nursing the cardiac parent and spouse back to health. You will all end up resenting it. Don't allow yourself to "out-think" the needs of your cardiac parent(s). Instead, sit down and talk with them, find out what their needs are from them, and after talking with your partner, decide what kind of help you can realistically offer. You can also elicit help from others in the family of from friends. Be the coordinator if you wish, but not the sole caretaker.

CHAPTER FIVE

DOCTORS AND NURSES

The cardiac patient presents a complex array of psychological symptoms, many of which complicate the recovery process and, in some cases, undermine attempts at medical treatment. Most patients suffer some depression and anxiety. When these symptoms become exaggerated, they can easily further complicate cardiac problems, whether real or perceived.

Psychotherapists address the patient's emotional concerns as they arise during the recovery process. Unfortunately, counseling should begin when the patient is first released from the hospital. And the person to whom the patient is most likely to turn for this is his doctor or nurse. Although these people are properly educated and trained on the medical side of heart disease, they are not always trained on the emotional side.

This chapter addresses some of the concerns that doctors and nurses may have about how to approach cardiac patients. I am routinely asked by the medical staff, "How can I help with the patient's emotional needs?" To those people, I hope the following information can be of some use.

Cardiac Profile

The recovering cardiac patient typically feels as though he's lost all control over himself and his environment, which comes from an overwhelming sense of helplessness. Confusion and fear of the future only complicate the situation. His moods may swing from one extreme to the other. He first must learn to come face-to-face with his illness and his emotions. At first, he will go into denial. Then his deep sense of inadequacy and dependency will yield guilt, frustration and a high degree of anger. Additionally, his self-esteem is at an all-time low. Put all these feelings together and it really becomes more than any one person can handle. Ultimately, he becomes more needy and clingy, and eventually his identity suffers.

Usually, the coronary patient has little tolerance for life's little wrinkles. He becomes selfish and insensitive to others. Most of the people around him are too busy telling him what to do, instead of just listening. A recent study (by the medical industry) revealed that cardiac patients most value a good listener and advice from a qualified medical doctor. The study further stated that doctors and nurses offer little, if any, psychological support for patients. Yet these are the people who can be most influential with their patients.

First Encounter

Whether you're a physician, nurse or psychotherapist, your relationship with the patient is usually grounded in your first encounter. Empathy, rapport, understanding and a caring attitude must be conveyed to the patient during this meeting. He needs to feel strength from your approach, and he needs to

71

know it's coming from a caring position. He also has to have confidence in your ability to help him.

Obviously, this is a lot to convey during a first encounter. And there are many approaches you can take with a cardiac patient. A lot depends on the patient's personality and temperament. Here is the approach I typically use when meeting a patient for the first time.

DOCTOR

I already have your age and I know a little about the medical side of things from your doctor. But I'd like you to tell me about your heart attack and what you're going through.

PATIENT

I had been having chest pains for awhile. My chest felt tight. I just passed it off as stress or something I had eaten. I guess I should have gone to the doctor.

DOCTOR

Most cardiac patients tend to ignore the symptoms. It's their way of denying the fact that there may be a problem as serious as a heart attack.

PATIENT

Maybe. At any rate, one afternoon the pain got worse. I felt nauseous. I had my secretary call 911. I was fairly convinced it was a heart attack.

DOCTOR

Has there been a history of heart disease in your family?

PATIENT

> *My father died of a heart attack, and two of my uncles. Because of them, I tried to read as much as I could about the symptoms of heart disease. I obviously didn't read it carefully.*

DOCTOR

> *You're being too hard on yourself. Most cardiac patients don't want to recognize the symptoms. It's called denial. Tell me more about your heart attack.*

PATIENT

> *When I got to the hospital, they told me I had suffered a heart attack. They did an angio-something or other and said I had three coronary arteries that had 'sufficient' blockage. One was completely blocked.*

DOCTOR

> *I have a good idea how you felt physically. But how did you feel emotionally at that point?*

PATIENT

> *I'm not sure. I know I was scared and confused. Everything happened so quickly. They told me I needed immediate bypass surgery. Even though my wife was there with me, I felt alone.*

DOCTOR

> *Most patients do at that point.*

PATIENT

> *They performed a quadruple bypass. They told me I was lucky because there was little damage to the heart. I didn't feel lucky. I hurt, physically and emotionally.*

> *Back in the hospital room, my wife started crying. I tried to hold back the tears.*

DOCTOR

> *What did **you** need at that point?*

PATIENT

> *I needed to hear from my wife that everything was going to be okay. I needed to know that I wasn't going to die.*

DOCTOR

> *Did you talk to her about your feelings?*

PATIENT

> *No.*

DOCTOR

> *Why not?*

PATIENT

> *I didn't want to upset her or scare her any further. She was frightened enough.*

DOCTOR

> *Maybe you didn't want to talk about it, either.*

PATIENT

> *That's a good possibility. It has been a month and I still don't want to talk about it.*

DOCTOR

> *What is it that you want from me?*

PATIENT

I guess someone who can understand what I'm going through and who can help me get back to work. It's hard to get motivated, and I'm extremely irritable and don't know why.

DOCTOR

Possibly because you're depressed and anxious about your future. We're talking about a deep sense of loss here, and it makes perfect sense that you would feel this way. You're also feeling confused.

Get yourself a notebook. You're going to have a lot of questions that need answers. Let's see if we can't answer some of them together.

COMMUNICATION

Cardiac patients have a tremendous need to communicate their experiences over and over again. To most health professionals, this may seem repetitive. But it's important that the patient be given an opportunity to expunge from his system this terrifying experience. It can serve as a catharsis, of sorts.

The health professional must learn to focus on the process of communication and not necessarily the content. For example, when your patient begins talking louder and faster about his sense of helplessness, he's really expressing his anger. Once you are able to discern his anger, it's okay to interrupt the story because you've addressed the underlying issue — anger. You can do so simply by saying "You sound very angry." You do have to listen to enough content, however, to discern the process. If your perception is wrong, the patient will correct you by telling you how he feels.

After you and the patient have discussed the anger and other underlying feelings, he will more than likely go on with his story. If he doesn't, simply ask him to continue.

Some cardiac patients are extremely withdrawn and reluctant to share their feelings. Communication may seem strained and rather one-sided. But you're still serving as a sounding board for the patient and giving him valuable information.

DOCTOR (PSYCHOTHERAPIST)
   Your cardiologist tells me that you're having some problems. What's this all about?

PATIENT
   I feel lousy, sometimes.

DOCTOR
   What do you mean by lousy?

PATIENT
   You know. Lousy. Awful.

DOCTOR
   Can you be a little more specific?

PATIENT
   I have pains in my chest and I feel lazy.

DOCTOR
   What kinds of pain? Is it only when you exercise?

PATIENT
   No, it's regular pain, on and off.

DOCTOR

   Have you told your cardiologist about this?

PATIENT

   What for? I'm sure its nothing serious. Besides, she's too busy.

DOCTOR

   I'm concerned for you. You seem so withdrawn that I'm afraid you're not addressing your needs. Your pain may be psychosomatic, but you need to have it checked by your physician for your own benefit. Never allow chest pains to go unattended. It could be serious.

   (The patient's process of avoidance and denial makes it difficult for him to communicate. Your understanding of this process should help you obtain information.)

PATIENT

   I know. You're right.

DOCTOR

   It also sounds to me as though you're mad at your cardiologist because she's not as available to you as you would like her to be. Tell her that you need more of her time, at this particular stage. Tell her that you're scared and that you need more information.

PATIENT

   I'm not sure I can do that. But I guess I should give it a try. It helps to know that you think I should do it, too.

Getting to Know Your Patient: Techniques for Communication

Most cardiac patients have a hard time confronting their doctors. Typically, it's because of a lack of confidence and low self-esteem. Even under the best of circumstances patients find their physicians intimidating. Help them get past this barrier. Although it may be time-consuming at first, ultimately you will spend less time with the patient because he has built an emotional connection with you — and that means a quicker recovery. One study, in fact, concluded that patients who were unfamiliar with the cardiac rehabilitation staff were five times as likely to die suddenly, thus getting to know your patient is extremely important.

Your approach as a health professional must be warm, personal and nurturing. Put yourself in the patient's emotional state of mind. What are the qualities you would like to see in a caretaker? Your tone and the way in which you deliver your message is an integral component of the communication process. Threats, lectures and a general authoritative posture only distances the patient. Become patient-focused. Granted, a certain degree of emotional distance is part of the job description, but it doesn't justify coming across as cold or removed.

There's a certain way of listening that makes the speaker feel as though he is being understood. One technique the listener can use is to visually connect with the speaker. In other words, give the speaker good eye contact in order to project a sense of caring. Here are some listening techniques you may want to try:

- *Probing* is used to find out more about what the speaker wishes to communicate. Use questions like, "How does that make you feel?" or "I'd like to know more about that";

- *Clarifying* reassures the speaker that you received his message. Use comments such as, "It sounds as if you're not pleased with your progress" or "So you're saying that cardiac rehabilitation is a lot of hard work";

- *Mirroring* reflects back to the speaker the message, "Yes, I understand what you're saying." A simple nod, however, won't do the trick. You need to convey your personal interest and concern verbally. Starting with the pronoun "I" makes a big difference;

- *Empathy* allows the speaker to feel as though the listener comprehends the emotional side of his words. This deep sense of caring and understanding is the foundation of trust, which is basic for any healthy relationship. Use comments such as, "I understand your frustration at not being able to control your work environment" or "I feel overwhelmed with your emotional turmoil."

It's also helpful to give the speaker a synopsis of what you heard verbally and noticed nonverbally. It lets him know that you were listening which, in the long run, will help to build a trusting relationship.

Listening skills are not difficult to learn, but it does take time to incorporate them into your practice. It will help your patients alleviate some of their confusion and anxiety, and it will help them through the medical crisis and cardiac rehabilitation program. Effective listening also will allow nurses more freedom to attend to the psychosocial issues of cardiac recovery, which will make for a more comprehensive treatment program and increase the patient's compliance.

Questions

Cardiac patients need to know that they're not going crazy. Since the heart attack, their entire world has been turned upside down. Their thoughts are interrupted by concerns of invalidism, surgery and death. They're looking desperately for a sense of "normality" in their lives.

When interviewing your patients, pay close attention to how they look. Do they look disheveled? Are they keeping themselves clean? These could be signs of depression. Their eating and sleeping habits may also indicate depression. *Be more concerned about what they don't tell than what they do.* Read between the lines. Trust your perceptions and focus on the patient's feelings — which provide the motivation for behavior.

More than likely the patient will experience some degree of depression, anxiety, frustration and anger. He may appear egocentric and be overly sensitive to his body's aches and pains. His memory may be impaired, which would make it difficult for him to concentrate. Explain to him that his feelings are perfectly "normal." This will go a long way in providing the patient some relief.

I have put together a list of questions that will help you approach the patient about his illness. These should also help you differentiate between what is organic and what is psychosomatic.

- *You seem anxious today. How does this affect your behavior?*

- *You must be uncomfortable being as anxious as you are. Tell me about it.*

- *I can't imagine what it must feel like to be as depressed as you are. Tell me about it.*

- *You sound angry. Talk to me about this.*

- *I sense your anger and imagine people are put off by it. How do you experience it?*

- *Do you experience any chest pain when you're angry or anxious?*

- *How is your family reacting to you? Are you concerned about your family's well-being?*

- *How has your heart attack affected your family?*

- *Do you resent the fact that someone else has to take care of you?*

- *Medical treatment is so expensive these days. Are you worried about your finances? (If you provide no more than an opportunity for catharsis, you've really helped.)*

- *You seem quiet today. Is anything wrong?*

OR

- *I'm not used to your being so quiet. What's wrong?*

- *You seem far away. Is anything bothering you?*

- *I find it difficult to connect with you today. Where are your thoughts?*

- *Tell me about your eating habits. Are you eating regularly?*

- *Your wife is concerned about your attitude towards eating. Is this a problem for you?*

- *I know you have a lot on your mind. I wonder if you're having trouble sleeping?*

OR

- *When I have things on my mind, I usually find it difficult to sleep. How about you?*

- *You look depressed, yet you say you're not. I'm concerned about this. Mind if we explore this area?*

Let's take one of these questions and plug it into a scenario between a doctor and his patient.

DOCTOR (CARDIOLOGIST)
    You seem quiet today. What's wrong?

PATIENT
    Everything. I don't know where to begin.

DOCTOR
    Any place you'd like.

PATIENT
    I've been feeling down, lately, and I don't know why. I'm doing well in my rehab program, and my physical exam came out okay.

DOCTOR
    So physically you're doing well. Emotionally, however, you're having some problems. That's a

natural reaction. You haven't been back to work yet, and I suspect you're questioning your ability to do so.

PATIENT

I'm questioning my ability to do anything. I want to take care of my family, but I'm not sure I can and I'm not sure I want to push myself.

DOCTOR

Sounds to me as though your values are changing somewhat.

PATIENT

Maybe. I'm not sure what I think, anymore. And I'm still worried that I'm not entirely healthy, although you say that I am.

DOCTOR

Cardiac patients typically perceive themselves that way. Your self-perception is distorted, which makes life more confusing and causes you to wonder if you'll ever be well.

PATIENT

So other cardiac patients feel the same way?

DOCTOR

Absolutely. But let's talk about you. I'm concerned about the way in which you handle your feelings. When something bothers you, you seem to withdraw from others. What you may not realize is that when you do this — suppress your emotions — you cause yourself more harm than good. I want you to start sharing these feelings with your wife and family. I think it'll help all of you.

Interactions with the Family

The cardiac spouse provides another dimension from which to observe the patient. An interview with the spouse often yields insight into the dynamics of heart disease. (Refer to Chapter Four for an in-depth perspective on the family dynamics of heart disease.)

Typically, it's not the patient but his family who create havoc with the medical and rehab staff. Obviously, they want the best possible treatment for their loved one. Anything less, will usually cause an uproar. In most cases, this kind of confrontation will elicit a defensive posture from the health care professional. It's hard to just brush off criticism. Yet I think it's imperative that you use their anger to attempt to close the emotional gap between yourself and the family. Do so by addressing the family's anger.

Family members need to be included in the treatment process. It helps them better understand the dynamics of heart disease from the patient's perspective. As roles change within the family unit, they will need to know how to adapt. As problems arise, they will need to know how to solve them together, not in isolation of the patient. More importantly, they will need to know how to handle their own emotions.

Doctors and nurses who work with cardiac patients must also address the psychosocial needs of the entire family. This may require in-house training and workshops. Through these efforts you should be able to teach family members how to address their own needs first, and then those of the patient.

With this goal accomplished, resentment will be kept to a minimum and everyone should be satisfied with the results.

NURSE

I'm concerned about the anger you've just expressed. Your need to feel this way makes sense. Perhaps I can help you through this difficult period.

WIFE

I'm just not myself. My husband was trying to get your attention, and he couldn't. Maybe I overreacted. I'm sorry.

NURSE

I think your reaction was the result of your frustration and sense of helplessness. I know it's hard on you, but your reaction is common among family members of cardiac patients. Your life has just been turned upside down. You're experiencing a tremendous loss and you're going to feel irritable and angry.

WIFE

Some mornings I just can't get out of bed. I feel tired and helpless.

NURSE

These are natural responses to the stress and depression. You're confused and anxious. When it reaches a boiling point you lash out, usually at the person who's closest to you — like your husband.

WIFE

>   *I am angry at him, but I'm afraid to upset him.*

NURSE

>   *I can understand why you'd feel this way. But I think you should know that your husband is not that fragile. His condition won't get worse just because you told him your feelings. As a matter of fact, by sharing your feelings you're actually creating an emotional bond, which will help improve his condition.*

WIFE

>   *Really? But he gets angry every time I get angry with him.*

NURSE

>   *There are different ways of dealing with anger. He's going to have to learn how to handle his anger and other feelings. Why don't we both help him find a way to express his emotions.*

WIFE

>   *If you think it would do some good.*

NURSE

>   *I do. By the way, a little emotional outburst is not necessarily a bad thing. It can help serve as a pressure valve.*

WIFE

>   *I can appreciate that. Thanks for the advice.*

NURSE

>   *We can talk again sometime. How about tomorrow?*

A short, concise conversation can do a great deal to diffuse a stressful situation. There may even come a time when you'll want to start a spousal support group. Just a few minutes a day can help the patient feel more at ease and make your task less stressful.

I'm Going Nuts! The Mental Well-Being of the Health Professional

A cardiac crisis can also greatly affect you, the health professional. As we all know, it's hard not to get emotionally attached to some patients. How do you cope with your own emotions, when you're busy comforting others? Obviously, your emotional well-being is just as important as the patient's. Some health professionals who experience job burn-out turn to drugs or alcohol.

Ideally, you should belong to a support group. It would provide you with a vehicle to vent your own feelings, and to receive feedback from your colleagues. Unfortunately, economic factors may prevent enrolling in an established group. Thus, one alternative is to start a support group of your own. Schedule meetings with your colleagues on a regular basis. Do it with up to 12 participants, but no more. If you can only get three that's okay, too. If you're fortunate enough to have surrounded yourself with a staff that you can trust, confide in these people. Use them as your support group. Find colleagues who are willing to help each other. There is no excuse to isolate yourself. The more you can share of yourself, the more available you can be to others.

CHAPTER SIX

OF A MEDICAL NATURE

COMMON QUESTIONS

Patients often ask me medical questions. What is a coronary artery bypass graft? What is an angiogram? Since I'm not a medical doctor, I typically refer these patients to their cardiologist. However, I do understand their need to have *all* of their questions answered. It helps relieve anxieties created by the many unknowns associated with heart disease.

This chapter, therefore, presents answers to some of the more frequently asked medical questions. This information serves only as a cursory note to the medical side of heart disease. It is not an exhaustive study by any means. Consult your physician for a more in-depth explanation.

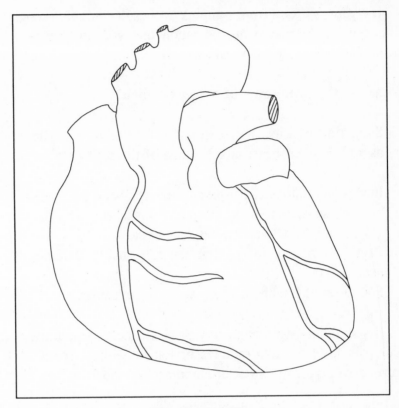

The Normal Heart

What is Angina Pectoris?

Angina is cause by a reduced flow of blood and oxygen to the heart, a condition known as ischemia. It usually occurs when the heart works harder than normal. You know you have it when you experience the following symptoms, which are similar in nature to the symptoms associated with a heart attack: intense discomfort, crushing pressure, squeezing or a burning sensation in the chest cavity (pectoris), and pain that may radiate to the arms, shoulders, back or neck. It may also be similar to what you would feel if you were suffering from indigestion.

If you suffer from angina, consult your physician immediately. Angina is an indication that you are at risk for cardiac problems, but it is *not* a heart attack.

What are the symptoms of a heart attack?

Symptoms of a heart attack may include all of the following or, as with a silent heart attack, none of the following:

- Intense discomfort, crushing pressure, squeezing or a burning sensation in the center of the chest. The pain will usually last two minutes or longer.
- Pain may radiate to right or left arm, back, shoulder, neck or jaw.
- Shortness of breath, nausea, sweating, dizziness.

If you should experience any or all of these symptoms, and your pain lasts for two minutes or longer without relief from rest or nitroglycerin, call your emergency number immediately.

What is hypertension?

Hypertension or high blood pressure is a condition whereby excessive pressure is directed on the inner walls of the arteries.

As your heart contracts and pumps blood through the arteries, pressure is created. If your blood pressure is higher than 140 over 90, you are suffering from hypertension, which may contribute to heart attacks, strokes, and atherosclerosis.

What causes high blood pressure (hypertension)?

The causes of high blood pressure are mostly unknown. However, overweight people and people who have a high-salt

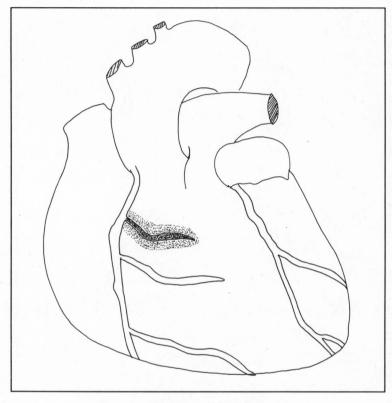

Heart with Myocardial Infarction

diet are likely candidates. Older people and those with a family history of heart problems are more susceptible to high blood pressure. Thus, age and heredity are two contributing factors.

What is a myocardial infarction?

Myocardial infarction — or "heart attack" as most people know it — occurs when the blood supply to the heart is interrupted for 20 minutes or more, which causes the affected part of the heart muscle to die.

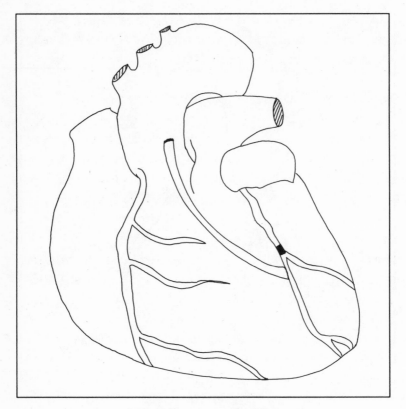

Artery Bypass to the Heart

What is coronary artery bypass graft (CABG)?

CABG (or coronary artery bypass surgery) is an operative procedure used to bypass an obstruction or blockage in one or more of the coronary arteries. Typically a vein from the leg or chest is used to reroute the flow of blood, oxygen and nutrients. The original artery is left intact.

What is coronary artery disease?

Coronary artery disease (CAD) is another term for "hardening of the arteries" (arteriosclerosis). It is also referred to as coronary heart disease (CHD).

What are arteriosclerosis and atherosclerosis?

Arteriosclerosis is a progressive disease more commonly known as "hardening of the arteries." Actually, the artery walls become thicker and less pliable, making them more susceptible to a build up of fatty substances known as cholesterol. Other fats also contribute to this build up. This process, it is believed, begins in childhood and may take 30 or more years to affect the arteries in such a way as to make them partially or totally blocked. This is known as atherosclerosis, which is a form of arteriosclerosis. When the coronary arteries reach this level of occlusion, a heart attack can occur.

Although the body naturally manufactures its own cholesterol, and is found in every cell in the body, certain foods like egg yolks, poultry, red meat, fish and whole milk dairy products can increase cholesterol levels. It is imperative to monitor your diet.

What is an angiogram?

An angiogram is a procedure used to detect coronary arteries that are closed off to one degree or another due to plaque build-up. During an angiogram, a catheter (plastic tube) is inserted into an artery in the groin or arm and passed through to the heart. Dye is injected and x-rays are taken at various points along the way. This helps doctors detect narrowed passages.

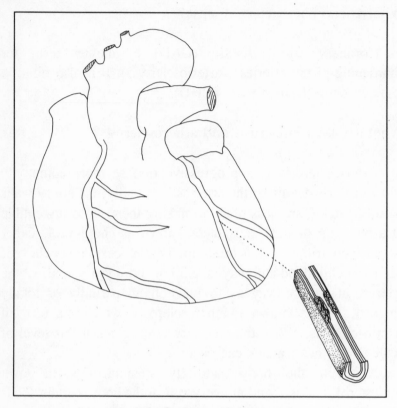

Partial Blockage of the Artery

What is angioplasty?

Once narrowed areas of the coronary artery are pinpointed by means of an angiogram, another catheter with a deflated balloon attached to its tip is inserted into an artery in the groin. The balloon is moved to the narrowed portion of the artery and inflated in an attempt to flatten the fatty deposits on the interior walls of the artery. This procedure usually takes about an hour, and carries some degree of risk, so you must understand all of the implications of this procedure. Most patients leave the hospital in 24-48 hours.

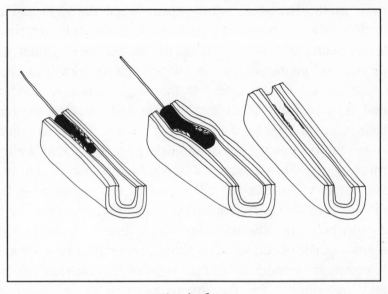

Angioplasty

What exactly does the heart do?

The heart is an organ about the size of two fists that pumps roughly 1,800 gallons of blood per day through 12,400 miles of arteries, veins and capillaries. It functions as a four-chambered pumping system.

How does the four-chambered pumping system work?

Actually, there are four separate pumps, together just a bit larger than your fist. The two chambers located at the top are known as the atria, and the two chambers located on the bottom are known as the ventricles. This magnificent "machine" is kept in proper cadence by an electrical impulse, which contracts each chamber in succession. Four valves allow the blood to flow in the proper direction. Between the right atrium, where the pumping process begins, and the right ventricle, there is a valve

95

known as the tricuspid, which opens when the right atrium contracts to allow blood to pass through to the right ventricle. As this ventricle contracts, it opens another valve called the pulmonic or pulmonary valve, which allows blood to flow through the pulmonary artery to the lungs. It is here that the blood relieves itself of carbon dioxide and takes on oxygen, which makes it bright red in color. It's journey now continues through the pulmonary veins, ultimately emptying into the left atrium, which when contracted sends blood through the now open mitral valve into the all important left ventricle — the main pump of the heart. The left ventricle has accountability to the entire body, because when contracted it sends blood through the now opened aortic valve to the entire circulatory system.

You might wonder about the origin of the electrical current that is responsible for the rhythmic action of the heart. It originates in a highly-specialized collection of cells in the right atrium. It is known as the sinoatrial node and is triggered by impulses from the brain.

What are arrhythmias?

Arrhythmias are irregularities in the normal rhythm of the heart. They have an electrical origin and can be treated with drugs or an artificial pacemaker.

Ventricular tachycardia or ventricular fibrillation, two types of arrhythmias, can be treated with a defibrillator, which sends an electrical shock to the heart, in an attempt to correct the electrical impulse. If your heart frequently goes into fibrillation, your doctor may order you to have a portable defibrillator available or have one implanted. Arrhythmias can cause death within a few minutes. Contact your physician immediately if you experience irregular beats.

Is medication available that can help prevent my coronary arteries from becoming blocked again?

This question is best answered by your physician. However, there are medications available by prescription only that help reduce the amount of cholesterol in your blood, thereby slowing the rate of atherosclerosis. With marked lowering of cholesterol, reversal of this process has been demonstrated. Additionally, there is some promising research that focuses on aspirin as a cholesterol reducing agent that is yielding positive results.

Your best approach is to stick to a low-fat, low-cholesterol diet, quit smoking and start exercising. You're going to have to work at keeping your arteries clear of deposits.

Information about the drugs that are prescribed for you can be confusing and difficult to understand. The pharmaceutical information in the following sections should make it easier for you to learn more about your medications. It appears courtesy of Cardiac Rehabilitation at Torrance Memorial Hospital in Torrance, California.

HEART MEDICATIONS

Anticoagulants

Types	Warfarin (Coumadin, Panwarfin)
	Ticlid (Ticlopidine)
Basic	
Action	Lengthens the time it takes for blood to clot.
Uses	For blood thinning, or to prevent blood clots.
Side	Prolonged bleeding time, nausea, vomiting,
Effects	bloating, gas, diarrhea, rash, hemorrhage with
	excessive dosage.

General Information: At first, frequent blood tests will be necessary to judge the drug's effectiveness.

Take medication at the same time each day. Do not stop taking the medication without consulting your physician.

Your skin may bruise more easily with anticoagulants. Contact your physician if any of the following danger signs occur: bleeding, coughing up blood, or large, severe bruises.

If you cut yourself, immediately apply firm pressure. If the bleeding does not stop within several minutes, call your physician.

Consult your physician before you start any other drugs, including non-prescription drugs, particularly those containing aspirin.

Cholesterol Lowering Agents

Types   Cholestyramine (Questran)
Clofibrate (Atromid — S)
Colestipol (Cholestid)
Gemfibrozil (Lopid)
Lipitor (Atarvostatin)
Lescol (Fluvastatin)
Lovastatin (Mevacor)
Niacin (Nicobid)
Pravachol (Pravastatin)
Zocor (Simvastatin)

Basic   Combines with bile acids to form an insoluble
Action   compound that is excreted from the body.
Inhibits production of cholesterol.

Uses   For elevated cholesterol and/or triglyceride levels.

Side   Nausea, vomiting, diarrhea or constipation,
Effects bloating, gas, rash, flushing of the skin.

General Information: Cholesterol levels will be checked one to two months after starting medication to evaluate effectiveness.

Take with meals to minimize stomach upset.

Aspirin

Types   Anacin
Ascriptin
Bayer
Bufferin
Ecotrin
Excedrin

Basic Action	Decreases the adhesiveness of the blood. This helps to prevent blood clots from forming in your arteries.
Uses	Before or after a heart attack. After coronary artery bypass graft surgery.
Side Effects	Prolonged bleeding time, ringing in the ears, nausea, vomiting, diarrhea, rash.

General Information: Take with food, milk, antacid or large glass of water to reduce side effects.

Daily doses are prescribed for the blood clotting effect, not for the relief of pain. If you need a pain reliever for headache, fever, etc., consult your physician.

Nitrates

Types	Nitroglycerin (NTG, Nitro-Bid, Nitro-Dur, Nitrostat) Imdur & ISMO Monoket (Isosorbide Mononitrate) Isosobide Dinitrate (Isordil, Sorbitrate) Erythrityl Tetranitrate (Cardilate) Pentaerythritol Tetranitrate (Peritrate)
Basic Action	Expands blood vessels which increases oxygen and blood flow to the heart, slight decrease in blood pressure.
Uses	Angina (chest pain) Congestive heart failure (CHF) Heart attack
Side Effects	Dizziness, especially with a change in body position, headache, rash with use of skin patches, weakness.

General Information: Dissolve sublingual tablets under the tongue. Don't chew or swallow.

Keep tablets in original, closed container. They will lose their potency if not kept in air-tight container.

Write date on bottle as soon as opened. Medication is generally good for three to four months after opening.

Sublingual tablets should produce a tingling sensation. If not, they have lost their potency.

Antiarrhythmic Agents

Types	Quinidine
	Procainamide (Pronestyl)
	Disopyramide (Norpace)
	Lidocaine
	Phenytoin (Dilantin)
	Tocainide (Tonocard)
	Mexiletine (Mexitil)
	Flecainide (Tambocor)
	Bretylium (Bretylol)
	Amiodarone (Cordarone)
	Digoxin
	Encainide (Enkaid)
Basic Action	Normalizes the heart's rate of contraction. Increases the heart's pumping efficiency.
Uses	To correct irregular heart rhythm, and some types of very rapid heart rates.
Side Effects	Can make the rhythm abnormality worse, nausea, vomiting and diarrhea, loss of energy, confusion, lightheadedness, depression, headache, hypertension, and lower heart rate.

General Information: If you notice an increase in palpitations, rapid heart rate or fainting, call your physician immediately.

Have your physician or pharmacist review all of your medications to guard against drug interactions. Check with your physician or pharmacist before starting on any over-the-counter medication.

Calcium Channel Blockers

Types
Cardene (Nicardipine)
Ditiazem (Cardizem, Cardizem CD, Dilicor XR, Tiazac)
Dynacirc (Isradipine)
Nifedipine (Procardia, Adalat)
Norvasc (Amlodipine)
Plendil (Felodipine)
Sular (Nisoldipine)
Verapamil (Isoptin, Calan)

Basic Action
Decreases the amount of calcium into the arteries. This prevents narrowing of the arteries, and reduces blood flow.

Uses
Hypertension (high blood pressure)
Angina (chest pains)
Irregular heart rhythms

Side Effects
The following are generally not serious and rarely require discontinuation of therapy: arm and leg swelling, dizziness, light-headedness, headache, nausea and flushing.

General Information: Have your physician or pharmacist review all of your medication to guard against drug reactions.

Beta Blockers

Types   Atenolol (Tenormin)
Acebutolol (Sectral)
Betaxolol (Kerlone)
Bisoprolol (Zebeta)
Carteolol (Cartrol)
Carvedilol (Coreq)
Esmolol (Brevibloc)
Labetalol (Normodyne or Trandate)
Metoprolol (Lopressor)
Nadolol (Corgard)
Penbutolol (Levatol)
Pinctolol (Visken)
Propranolol (Inderal)
Sotalol (Betapace)
Timolol (Blocadren)
Toprol XL (Metoprolol)

**Basic
Action**   Slows heart rate and decreases blood pressure.

Uses   Angina
Hypertension
Antiarrhythmic effect (irregular heart beats)
Myocardial infarction (to decrease the workload
of the heart)

**Side
Effects**   Decreased energy, decreased exercise tolerance,
shortness of breath, dizziness, sleep disturbances,
impotence and slightly clouded sensorium

General Information: Do not stop taking medication unless instructed by your physician. It can be dangerous to stop the medication abruptly.

ACE Inhibitors

Types   Benazepril (Lotensin)
              Catopril (Capotan)
              Enalapril (Vasotec)
              Fosinopril (Monopril)
              Lisinopril (Prinivil, Zestril)
              Moexipril (Univasc)
              Quinipril(Accupril)
              Ramipril (Altace)

Basic   Decreases blood pressure and reduces resistance for
Action   pumping action of the heart.

Uses   Hypertension
              Congestive Heart Failure

Side   Dry, non-productive cough
Effects

General Information: Consult physician before stopping medication or when using with other medications.

CHAPTER SEVEN

CARDIAC RECOVERY PROCESS

Most patients associate cardiac recovery with physical exercise and the healing of an organic medical condition. But full recovery requires both a healthy body and a sound mind. Time spent in a cardiac recovery program (typically about three months) is only the beginning of a new lifestyle. *Your psychological well-being is the foundation from which you can strengthen your physical self.*

The psychological components of heart disease (i.e., emotions, attitudes, self-concepts) and a high degree of self-awareness, help hold together the other two elements of cardiac recovery (exercise and the medical condition). All three must work together as a well-oiled machine. If there's a glitch, you will be frustrated in your efforts to recover.

The recovery process begins with the first signs of heart disease. Your mind reviews all the possibilities: death, invalidism, physical limitations, and so on. The recovery process is different for each individual, depending upon their life experiences, and basic psychodynamics (their own personal psychology). However, the following basic phases are frequently experienced and are common enough to be applied to most cardiac patients. (Please refer to Recovery Process chart on facing page.)

Your physician may be able to provide you with some degree of comfort by clarifying the many unknowns associated with heart disease. A better understanding of your condition will help you deal with the physical and emotional dynamics.

The second phase of the recovery process represents the impact of a cardiac event on your attitude. Included are the emotions that yield to a lowered sense of self esteem and may impact your identity as you once knew it.

In phase III your behavior is clearly a manifestation of your feelings and attitude, and is indicative of your fear, insecurity and helplesness. It is also the time during which you enter cardiac rehabilitation to build both emotional and physical strength.

After increased self-confidence because of your experience with cardiac rehab, Phase IV begins to reflect your new emerging sense of self and perhaps most importantly your ability to handle such changes. (Allow about three months for this period, as indicated in the chart. It will take time for your altered self-concept to catch up to your changes in behavior.) You are, in fact, changing your lifestyle, and Phase V points out the many facets and complexities of such a transition.

Finally in Phase VI, you can begin to emerge with an altered sense of self. Many changes are still to come, but now

SIX PHASES OF EMOTIONAL CARDIAC REHABILITATION (Six months to a year)

PHASE I
Initial Impact of Cardiac Disease

ISSUES: Who Am I? (Self-Concept Shattered)
Panic
Fear
Confusion
Unknowns
Will I Live/Die?
Disability
Invalidism

PHASE II
Attitudinal Changes

ISSUES: Self Pity (Why Me?)
Narrowed Self Concept
Negative Thinking
Confusion
Fear and/or Anxiety
Depression
Anger → Rage
Low Self Esteem
Identity Issues
Egocentricity

PHASE III
Behavioral Changes

ISSUES: Isolation
Over-activity
Aggression
Withdrawal
Physical Limitations
Hard to be with
Cardiac Rehabilitation

(3 Months)

PHASE IV
Altered Self-Concept

ISSUES: Thoughts
Ideas
Values
Patterns of Relating
Fear of Unknown
What am I becoming?
Increased Self-confidence

PHASE V
Lifestyle Changes

ISSUES: Patterns of Relating
Diet
Occupations
Work Patterns
Leisure Time
Risk Factor Modification
Exercise
Trial and Error

PHASE VI
Becoming

ISSUES: Emotional Intimacy
Emerging Self-concept
Values and Ideas
Focus of Life
Clarity of Direction
Increased Self-Esteem
Cardiac Awareness
Health Consciousness

you are sensitive to other's needs and aware of what is important in life. Emotional intimacy and clarity of direction are keys for your continued emotional growth.

Naturally, we can't completely change our behavior. But we can make the necessary changes to affect the quality of our lives, which is the key issue for cardiac patients. As your self-concept improves, through behavioral changes, you'll find yourself relating to others differently. Your relationships will take on a new priority and meaning, which will make life more productive for you and your family.

The emotional connections you are able to build, as well as your lifestyle — which includes everything from diet to leisure time — are the keys to improving the quality of your life. As you walk down the path to recovery, your new sense of self-awareness, style of communication and emotional exposure will be reflected in everything you do.

BIBLIOGRAPHY

American Psychological Association, Inc. *Ethical Principles in the Conduct of Research with Human Participants*. American Psychological Association, Inc., Washington, D.C. 1973.

American Psychological Association, Inc. *Ethical Standards of Psychologists*. American Psychological Association, Inc., Washington, D.C. 1977.

Billings, R.F., Kearns, P.M., Levene, D.C. *Influence of Psychological Factors on Chest Pain Associated with Myocardial Infarction*. ACTA. Med. Scand. (suppl.), 1981.

Blackburn, H. "Risk Factors and Cardiovascular Disease." *The American Heart Association Heartbook: A Guide to Prevention and Treatment of Cardiovascular Diseases*. New York: Dutton, 1980

Boscaglia, Leo. *Loving Each Other: The Challenge of Human Relationships*. New York: Ballantine Books, 1984.

Brandenburg, R.O., McGoon, D.C. "Heart Valve Disease." *The American Heart Association Heartbook: A Guide to Prevention and Treatment of Cardiovascular Diseases*. New York: Dutton, 1980.

Bromburg, H., Donnerstag, E. "Counseling Heart Patients and their Families," *Health Social Work*, 177, Aug., 2(3), 158-172.

Cohn, Peter F. and Joan K. Cohn. *Heart Talk*. Orlando, Fla.: Harcourt Brace Jovanovich, 1987.

Collins, B. "Relationship Patterns Among Married and Unmarried Cohabitating Couples." *The Marriage and Family Counselors Quarterly*. 1978, Winter, 1-8.

Cousins, Norman. *Anatomy of an Illness*. New York: W.W. Norton & Company, Inc., 1979.

Cousins, Norman. *The Healing Heart*. New York: W.W. Norton & Company, Inc., 1979.

Croog, S.H., Fitzgerald, E.F. "Subjective Stress and Serious Illness of Spouse: Wives of Heart Patients." *Journal of Health and Social Behavior*. 1978, June, 19(2), 166-178.

Croog, S.H., Shapiro, D.S., Levine, S. "Denial Among Male Heart Patients: An Empirical Study." *Psychosomatic Medicine*. 1978, 33, 385-397.

Crouch, Michael A. and Conrad Roberts. *The Family in Medical Practice*. New York: Springer-Verlag. 1987.

Deracup, K.A., Breu, C.S. "Using Nursing Research Findings to Meet the Needs of Grieving Spouses." *Nursing Research.* 1978, July-August, 27(4), 212-216.

Foster, D.W. *A Layman's Guide to Modern Medicine.* New York: Simon & Schuster, 1980.

Friedman, M., Byers, S.O., Rosenman, R.H., Newman, R. "Coronary Prone Individuals (Type A Behavior Pattern), Growth Hormone Responses," *Journal of American Medical Association* 1971, 217, 929-932.

Friedman, M., Rosenman, R.H. *Type A Behavior and Your Heart.* New York: Fawcett Publication, 1974

Hampe, S.O. "Need of Grieving Spouse in Hospital Setting." *Nursing Research,* 1975, March-April, 24, 113-120.

Heath. "Myocardial Infarction: A Personal Account." *Journal of Rehabilitation.* 1966, March-April, 32, 2.

Jenkins, C.D. "Behavioral Risk Factors." *The American Heart Association Heartbook, A Guide to Prevention and Treatment of Cardiovascular Diseases.* New York: Dutton, 1980.

Kavanagh, S. "Sexual Activity After Myocardial Infarction." *Canadian Medical Association Journal.* 1977.

Likoff, W. "The Attack." *Journal of Rehabilitation.* 1966, March-April, 32, 2.

List, J.S. *A Psychological Approach to Heart Disease.* New York: Institute of Applied Psychology, 1967.

Lowen, Alexander. *God, Sex and Your Heart.* New York: MacMillan Publishing Co., 1988.

Maslow, A.H. *Toward a Psychology of Being.* New York: Litton Educational Publishing, Inc., 1968.

Mayou, R. "Course in Determinants of Reactions to Myocardial Infarction." *British Journal of Psychiatry,* 1979, June, 134, 588-594.

Mayou, R., Foster, A., Williamson, B. "Psychological and Social Effects of Myocardial Infarction on Wives." *British Medical Journal.* 1978, March, 1(6114), 699-701.

Medalie, J.H., Goldbourt U. "Angina Pectoris Among 10,000 Men. II Psychosocial and Other Risk Factors as Evidenced by a Multivariate Analysis of a Five Year Incidence Study." *American Journal of Medicine* 1976, May, 60(6), 910-21.

Parson T., Fox, R.C. "Illness and the Modern Urban Family." *Journal of Social Issues.* 1952, April, 13, 31-44.

Rossman, Martin L. *Healing Yourself.* New York: Pocket Books, A Division of Simon & Shuster, 1987.

Ryan, Regina and John W. Travis. *Wellness Workaholic*. Berkeley, CA: Ten Speed Press, 1981.

Schwartz, J. *Letting Go of Stress*. New York: Pinnacle Books, Inc., 1982.

Shepherd, J.T. "How the Heart Functions." *The American Heart Association Heartbook, A Guide to Prevention and Treatment of Cardiovascular Diseases*. New York: Dutton, 1980.

Shillingford, J.P. *Coronary Heart Disease*. New York: Oxford University Press, 1981.

Skelton, D. "Psychological Stress in Wives of Patients with Myocardial Infarction." *British Medical Journal*. 1973, 103.

Surwit, R.S., William, R.B. Shapiro, D. *Behavioral Approaches to Cardiovascular Diseases*. New York: Academic Press, Inc., 1982.

Szklo, M., Tonascia, Jr., Gordis, L. "Psychosocial Factors and the Risk of Myocardial Infarction in White Women." *American Journal of Epidemiology* 1976, March, 103(3), 312-320.

Viscott, David. *Risking*. New York: Pocket Books, A Division of Simon & Schuster, 1977.

Wenger, N.K. "Living with Cardiovascular Disease." *The American Heart Association Heartbook, A Guide to Prevention and Treatment of Cardiovascular Diseases*. New York: Dutton, 1980.

ABOUT THE AUTHOR

Dr. Herbert N. Budnick is a licensed psychotherapist who works almost exclusively with patients of heart disease and their families. He holds a Ph.D. in psychology.

For the past 12 years, Dr. Budnick has given workshops and seminars at hospitals and universities, and at local and state government agencies. His "Living with Heart Disease" lecture series and counseling programs — which are based, in part, on personal experience — have helped thousands of patients overcome the emotional disorders associated with heart disease.

Dr. Budnick lives in Southern California with his wife, Ceese.